CW01481046

The lion and the giant of my dreams

Maxene Hewitt

The lion
and the giant
of my dreams

An autobiography

Floris Books

First published by Floris Books, Edinburgh in 1987

© Ben Hewitt 1987
All rights reserved. No part of this publication may be reproduced
in any form without the prior permission of Floris Books, 21 Napier
Road, Edinburgh.

The publisher acknowledges subsidy from the Scottish Arts Council
towards the publication of this volume.

British Library CIP Data available

ISBN 0–86315–062–4

Printed in Great Britain
by Billings & Sons Ltd, Worcester

Contents

Presentiments   7

Prologue   9

1. The setting   11

A dream: The first meeting with the lion   17

2. "Buen"   19

3. The presage   24

4. April 7, 1943   27

A dream: The giant appears   32

5. Glimpses of silent fears   34

6. The terrifying tread of a giant recedes   42

7. An introduction   51

8. Adolescence   59

9. No wedding dress for me, please   68

10. The sun too has a shadow   72

11. The waning of my public eye   82

A contemplation: A look at blindness   99

12. Ben and Katie   100

13. A lump in my breast   108

A dream: A second meeting with the lion   115

14. Information from where?   116

15. The distant past   120

A dream: A third meeting with the lion   126

16. A critical reverie and meditation   127

17. Growing in new directions   131

18. Home again. Winter, June 1978   140

A dream: The last meeting with the lion   *148*

19. My mother's death   148

A dream: The mandala   *156*

20. Sylvia comes to rest. October 1980   157

A dream: Hiding the child away   *162*

21. The battle continues   163

22. Winter 1981   169

23. Isis   173

24. The passing of dark blood   179

25. The fire opens my eyes   181

A contemplation: My father beckons   *187*

26. The beginning of the end   188

27. Easter   195

A dream: My mother's voice   *203*

Poem   *205*

Postscript   207

Presentiments

I heard the crows again this morning. I hate crows. Anyone who has ever lived in the country hates crows. I hate crows. They attack tiny lambs — the defenceless children of God, they pick their eyes out — taking the life from their eyes before they die.

Crows are a symbol of untimely death — a black hole in a sunlit vista — a denial of Goodness overcoming Evil — an ever-present calling Caw, to be heard by a fearful and a materialistic mind.

I need a mystery; I need my spirit. You can hear me crying in the night, crying in the moonlight, away from the searing morning sun, crying with pain as my body seeks to bring forth my spirit here on Earth. Like the lamb, my eyes are blind, my breasts have been wrung and are dry, I cannot bear my fruit but my body screams out to reach its thwarted, full bloom, its ripeness, its fullness of life, its earthly ecstasy. My tears are not cleansing my body, or falling to warm the earth at my feet; they stream inwards like so many tiny, tense links in a chain to my death. Every linking drop is carrying a part of my Being, splashing into the quiet and silver formlessness of Eternity.

My arms reach to the yellow haze of the sun. Those crows cast a shadow on my pleading face to make a mockery of my strivings.

Prologue

Why didn't anyone hear me? Why didn't they hear me?

It was such a beautiful day. The day was filled with yellow sunshine. It was the kind of day so dense with golden light, that if an apple fell from its tree, it would be suspended in the rich fecundity of the air. This day's events changed the direction of my destiny — such an event should not have happened on such a day.

It happened when I went looking for my child. She was a bright, intelligent two-year-old with the prettiness of the young Goldilocks, who had never been walking in the woods. I can see us standing before the place — I had found my little one, playing there, picking wild flowers as yellow as the sun, quite oblivious of the moment. And so was I. There I was, the sleeves of my calico dress rolled up, bare legged, blossoming in full female beauty, knowing that I was loved, holding my daughter's hand, looking at a cellar door in the hillside.

The place looked deserted. I was drawn to that door as surely as one of those apples inevitably is drawn to the ground. I opened the door. Sun fell in a long slice of light across a decaying wooden floor. I dropped my daughter's hand. As I hesitated on the doorstep I noticed kegs in the corner and the moving stain of dark red wine which flowed from one of the dusky shapes. "Go home," I whispered, turning in the doorway, seeing for the last time the clear blue eyes of my cherished child who was already turning for flight, hugging the much loved form of her lifeless toy, whose blank, embroidered eyes stare at me still.

What could have drawn me to that place? What could have taken me, lured me from that happy life, those nights filled with the scent of first love, expressed in so many acts that are symbolic of joyous creativity, its movements echoing the pulsing of blood in bodies that are alive and alive and alive. Could the ecstasy, the climax of my perfect love, have drawn me to the pain, the darkness and the oblivion of my death — for I did die there, in the summer of my life — leaving the fruit of my healthy womb and the lean young man who had learnt with me the meaning of the words "flesh of one flesh". His arms had encircled me in pure nurture, his hair mingling with mine while we slept in peace every night of that life together.

How do the dead grieve their untimely parting? How do the dead say good-bye?

1. The setting

The small town where I was born lies on the side of a hill, a misshapen, sprawling square with roads like arms which meander into the ranges proper or back towards the arterial highways leading to the cities.

The house where I spent most of my early childhood was inside a corner of the square as you approached the town over the bridge from the south and just before the shops which were sprinkled among the houses on two sides of the square. Just as the roads echoed the line of the mountain stream, and the arcs of the mountain ridges, the small houses clung to the sides of the roads like leaves on the smaller branches of a tree. The head of the town nestled down into the river flats. The river was more precisely a creek and every season could be measured by its state. In summer it was a string of deep pools joined by ribbons of chocolate brown mud which dried in the sun and formed a crust to be walked on and broken through, revealing delicious warm ooze beneath. In some places a small trickle got through, running delicately over the stones and shale, carrying with it a few frogs' eggs, the tendrils and fluffs of green slime. It provided a moving footpath for the water spiders and a myriad of mirror images of the bright blue sky for the dragon-flies to hover above, their occasional darts of rapid flight making it appear as if they were trying to adjust the view of themselves in the water's face.

The end of summer came as a violent burst of electrical activity above the mountain peaks. Gone were the blanched tones of interminable heat in a few short hours; and gone were the droning sounds of a summer long. Cracks of golden light forked across the face of the upper sky as we fled inside to safety, with the sound of Thor's footsteps booming behind our running feet. As the light and rumblings reached an ecstatic state, with claps of thunder above our heads, the dark drifts of galleon cloud unleashed a deluge upon the shaken earth.

From our sunroom window, we watched the rain play out in miniature what was happening on a grander scale amongst the topmost peaks of the ranges. Pools appeared to overflow their edges, running rivulets to find their level in a torrent of gushing gutter or storm-filled drain.

As soon as the storm passed on, the word would run about that the river was running again. What magic method of telepathy told us this, I never discovered. With the first few drops of rain, we had drunk in the steaming smell of freshly washed earth, and now as the veil of summer dust was washed from leaves to ground, we saw the first colours of dark and watery winter. Down to the bridge we ran, jostling bareheaded in our rubber boots and coats for the spot marking the centre of the river's course. Sometime during an alert silence, we would hear the approach of the flash flood. At last it would appear around the bend — a huge wall of grumbling water, bringing with it a layer of rich brown dirt, washed from the dry breasts of the hills. It carried a debris of fallen branches and bodies, and along with them, the young green shapes of trees whose hold on the eroded banks of the dry creek bed had not been strong enough. We watched the rumbling and bobbing of discarded material possessions, probably thrown out after the buying fervour that Christmas brings. Old livestock who had clung close to the water holes during summer, were swept off their aged legs before their ears and nostrils registered the coming of the waters. Other glazed eyes and rigid carcasses floated past, accompanied by thousands of minute creatures in the muddy midst of that carrion flood.

The road over the bridge forked left to the cattle track and past the front of our shop to become the main street, Branscombe Street, the only road in the district with a tarred surface. In the hot summer sun we rode our bikes over its boiling bubbles, sending tiny black spots into the faces of our friends behind.

My father's sister lived opposite us with her family. At one stage she was almost in disgrace for she married a "Mick"; that is, a Roman Catholic. Pop and Ma King, my father's parents and members of long respected district families, lived next to us. They were fine, upstanding members of the Protestant community. Pop worked next door on the other side in Kellet's, the largest department store in the town. It had an imposing edifice of about a dozen steps leading to their show-room windows, but no one seriously used them, preferring to enter the store by the service entrance. Instead the steps were left to the leg-lifting dogs, running-up-and-down-children and the town's retired tramp. Old Ted sat in the alcove, a derelict figure, collating his fag ends and drinking from a bottle that seemed to materialize from nowhere. There he sat almost all day, out of the wind or the sun and on the edge of life. Just after I started school someone noticed that the steps seemed strangely empty and that Old Ted had not been seen for some time. My best friend's dad, Phil Orth, went to look for him. He found the old man on his bed of rags beneath the tank-stand on the edge of the oval where he lived. He was black with death and dirt, already decomposing, his body half-eaten by scavenging rats.

On the last corner of this shopping street sat the tiny Post Office building, also in sandstone where my parents worked together on what was for them both, their first jobs. My father did night-shift switchboard, the telegraph and Morse code work, while my mother did day-shift switchboard and was a nineteen-thirties version of the Post Master's girl Friday. My mother boarded with Auntie Annie on the hill. She was only eighteen when she started, but even so young, she was proud of being the trustee of so many town secrets which came to her ears, her eyes and through her hands.

Zena and Max courted in the first motor bike and side-car in the district. When they married in 1935, she was barely twenty, and my father little more. He gave her the first washing machine seen in these parts and managed to drive us round in a smart new family car, a Whippet, before he was off to the War.

My parents were members of the eager new era, but those machines that could have brought them freedom, also carried them into the world's melting pot where powerful men were to rearrange the patterns of our lives and change the direction of our faces in the future.

I was born when my parents lived next to the

bush nursing hospital on the hill. My mother simply crawled through the wire fence as soon as her first pains started at one o'clock in the morning, while Aunty Vera held the wires apart and held her case. My mother puffed a lot to keep me back at the last minute until the family doctor arrived from a trip up country to assist my delivery at 6.30 am. Mum was inundated with gifts for her first-born baby girl. Aunty Pearle (that was my mother's second name) hurried off to tell everyone that Mrs Maxie King has had a daughter and they've called her Magazine Annie. Poor Aunty Pearle was in her dotage. Her garbled version did not stop my name becoming Maxene (a combination of Max and Zena) but it did alter my parents' choice of Annie to the popular Shirley of those times. Anne would have been much more my choice. Shirley seems cheap, fussy and girlish in a way that has never suited what I wanted to be.

After my brother Brett was born we moved to Yoevil, a tiny town in the hot middle west. My mother often retold how she simply sat with Brett and me next to a baby bath full of water, during a ten-day century-heatwave, dunking us frequently and plying us with drinks.

From 1939 to the summer of 1948 I played on the cattle track which ran up the side of the hill beside our house. There I saw herds of sheep and cattle going north for agistment or south to escape the droughts; I saw families drive past with all their belongings stacked on the tray of a single truck and, more vividly still, armies of men, machines and lorries preparing for war. The cattle track was our filthy race track. Here my two brothers, Brett and

Graeme, and I learned to ride our first scooters, our first two-wheelers no hands, and it was here that I rode over the edge in my little red pedal car, to lie among the boulders a grazed and bloody mess. We came to no serious harm here but this track was so steep that travellers who knew the road, gradually speeded up as they came over the bridge so they did not conk out half-way up. It went for half a mile straight up the range to turn left on to the ridge road that led to my mother's parents' farm. Buen lay on the shoulder of the Black Range in the Great Divide. It was a beautiful location which looked out over the valleys and hazy blue rolling hills. It was here in the eye of the Sunburnt Country, that the heart of my childhood beat. Here dirty tufts of shed wool glistened with morning droplets like diamonds, and miniature wild flowers of palest blue tinkled the songs of a thousand years in my childish ears. The earth crackled and moved beneath my feet and before my eyes, veils of moving colours changed with the seasons. The sky was an eternity of spacious blue, dappled from time to time with drifts of tinted cloud which sometimes travelled slowly and distantly in the heavens, or descended low, throwing swift, dark shadows on the ground where I stood. There was nothing mean or wilful, nothing evil-doing, in that landscape I saw as a child. My grandparents inhabited it in the quiet certainty of its fertile goodness and in the aura of their vision, I saw it that way too.

Whenever people ask me about my childhood, I always describe it as idyllic. The setting of my early years was definitely idyllic — it was the drama of events that was not.

A dream: The first meeting
with the lion

*Around under the orange tree, where the air was like a
tender umbrella of perfume, I looked at the steepness of
the parapet above me. It was a long low wall which
ran the length of the verandah just outside my bedroom
and almost my height off the ground. Here was a piece
of isolated and unloved garden. I looked with great
speculation at the long spears of young spring grass
which had been allowed to grow to their full height. In
the orchard they would have been ploughed under when
they were only half this age, but here, the overflow of
water from the tended parts of the garden had been
drunk long and full, by their roots. I approached the
grass, wanting to throw myself full length into it,
thinking of it as a high, all-enveloping bed — a bed
just grown for the delight of a child, like me. With the
anticipation of an eager and trusting two-year-old, I
threw myself into it, but beneath the long strands lay
the earth that had become hard. It hadn't been touched
by fork or spade for years and had formed a thick crust.
The tall bed of soft grass had been an illusion and here
I was lying in its midst, knowing that when I stood its
call would be broken, its strands no longer able to stand.*

*I lay there looking up through the pattern of the
orange tree leaves, into the soft sky which was saying
goodbye to the sun's rays. As the blue dissolved, all
around me grew greyish green with the approaching*

shadow of the night. I turned my head and peered through the tiny fence of remaining strands of grass at the tree that I called the snowball tree. It had frail feathery leaves and minute marshmallowy balls, softer and smaller than lilypillies. The little balls were like a faint tracery of differing shadow. Beneath it, looking as though he had always been there, was a lion, a young, proud lion. We looked at each other, acknowledging each other's presence. We were both young. I was not exactly afraid, but I was full of respect. I stood up in what had been a miniature forest, and watching the lion all the way, I walked along the path past him, whilst he looked the other way like a cat who pretends not to see the bird.

As I came through the door from the front verandah, with interest and no anxiety (for I was inside) I said, " 'Dad," to my grandfather, "there's a lion in the garden."

"A lion!" he said. The disbelief in his voice was quickly overtaken by his acknowledgement of my fantasy world. Just in case it was no fantasy, and to do as I wanted, he went out to investigate.

"It truly was a lion," I said as he went down the steps and around the corner. I sat down in his chair, waiting. Now as I remember it, I wonder where my grandmother was. I was not afraid but sat there, a mute part of the first instalment of many encounters; for the lion would grow in my dreams as I would grow in my life.

Next I remember my grandparents reading their papers by the fire on that cool late spring evening. The colour of the sun lay round the kerosene lamp and now the shadows were warmed by the light and sound of our group.

"There hasn't been a circus in town for some time, and I haven't heard of one hereabouts. You must have been imagining it," said 'Dad. But in my memory it lies not as a dream but as a reality in another part of my being.

2. "Buen"

I cry when I read that word; I cry when I think of that place. "Buen" — a child's paradise; the place where all my childhood love sprang from, the place where all perfection was manifest.

My grandmother had created a garden there that glowed, that breathed life that you could drink in through your senses. A place where trees and shrubs and flowers grew which made you feel tenderness flow into your fingertips as you touched their fragile changing bodies. At night the garden spiders would fling themselves into the weaving of their webs. In the day the birds would sing and fly about their habitat, and under every fallen leaf and nestling stone, minute creatures carried out their incessant tasks.

As I look back and remember Buen, I experience it as a series of vignettes, edited so heavily that it lies like a perfect film in my memory. I remember sitting in the sulky with 'Dad, my beloved grandfather, breaking into the sunshine from the trees in the common and seeing the red roof of Buen blinking in the sun waiting for me; its windows looking out from beneath the hood of its surrounding verandahs. At its feet a lucerne patch lay, gently moving, a soft shadow, a purple haze of lucerne blooms. My memories exist beyond the realms of time, of sequence and of logic.

As I remember it the dogs still bark at our approach.

As we pulled up I would hear the back wire-screen door slam shut, and there Auntie Vera would be, laughing and talking all at once, ready to receive me as 'Dad lifted me out of the sulky in a great arc of happy movement. From the arms of one loved person into the caring hands of another I would pass.

On we would go under the archway of wistaria which hung over our heads as we walked from the back gate towards the noisy activity of the farm kitchen.

There in the kitchen, my grandmother was creating foods and an atmosphere of a different kind. Like the central character of a play, there she would be, orchestrating all activity, creating a world fit for those she loved. There she always was, with open arms. It was only when I was in those arms talking with her, surrounded by all she had brought to our world, that I felt I was really home; for this was where I belonged, this was my heart's home.

Soon I would be running along the paths which bordered three sides of the house. These paths were lined with old-fashioned flowers just made for the delight of a child. There were violets who drink through their flower faces and whose lives would end too quickly if their stems were crushed by over-enthusiastic fingers. What a long time it took me to pick a bunch big enough to take inside when I only had the tiniest too-careful fingers of a breathless child. In that garden I exchanged long ardent looks with the intent upturned faces of the pansies as I passed them by. Hen and chicken plants, and agapanthus stood by my side. Snapdragons, cosmos, larkspurs, poppies and so many flowerheads of bobbing colour fill my memory, that now my head almost bursts with the memory of it all.

Sometimes during the day of each new visit Grandma and I would water the garden together, inspecting new flowers, investigating the staghorns to see if any new buds were nestling in its middle, and together we would visit the fernery. This visit was by special dispensation, for children normally were not allowed in this place where Grandma nursed seeds into life, seedlings into strong growth, and protected plants and flowers who could not survive in the harsh outer world.

As the sun was setting I would join Grandad in his round of feeding and watering the animals and birds. There was wheat to be ground, hens and chicks to be lured into the fowlhouse, dogs to be fed and watered and chained up for the night, and finally the kindling and wood prepared for overnight fires.

That night by the fire I would listen to 'Dad playing the Jew's harp which lived inside the Ansonian clock on the mantelshelf. Almost asleep in my grandmother's arms I could watch the firelight continuously altering the light and shade in the room, releasing and hiding the colours and shapes while I slipped in and out of waking and dreaming, revelling in the moment of security and pleasure and planning the following day, knowing that it would be as perfect as ever. I would finally drift into sleep in the midst of a mass of feathery eiderdown and pillow, listening to the clock in the loungeroom next door tick-tocking in its regular predictable rhythm and the gentle voices of the three people who would help me to fashion the following day. Of course my mind tells me that I didn't always sleep in my grandparents' bed, but in my memory it is the best place to be.

My most special time with 'Dad was to accompany him on his rounds of the sheep. He would tie a pillow to the pommel of the saddle and off we would go, with me sitting on the pillow and with 'Dad holding me and an umbrella in his left hand (just in case the sun was too hot for my head) and with the reins firmly held in his right hand.

Sometimes in the heat of the day I would escape to the orchard, for this was the only place I could truly be alone. I mostly remember the delicious taste of sun-warmed peaches and apricots, plums and nectarines.

"Not too many at once. Don't eat them while they're still green," Grandma would warn me from the other side of the fence.

The orchard was paradoxically not only the place where heavenly gifts seemed close at hand, but it was also the place of two painful memories. A bee sting is a common thing in the life of a country child, but to experience it for the first time on the sensitive lobe of your ear while you are busily engaged in eating a luscious globe of golden fruit, didn't seem to be right.

On another occasion when still very young, I tried

to peer into the home of newly-hatched birds and in the process I scratched myself badly and saw with horror that I had knocked a sleeping featherless baby bird out of its nest and on to the harsh ground at the foot of the tree. The pinky grey flesh of the baby bird showed its rapidly beating heart all too clearly to my devastated gaze. Now as I try to recall the outcome of that incident in the orchard, my childhood shock draws a curtain across my consciousness.

There are many revelations in childhood which bring a balance of shadow to the light. At Buen the darker sides, the more dangerous sides of nature were dealt with simply and without fuss. On Monday mornings when the copper was lit for the week's wash, a rolled up newspaper was first lit and pushed into the firebox to flush out the deadly red-backed spiders. It seems odd to me now that the time and place I associate with the richest and happiest part of my childhood, was also potentially the most dangerous. Actually besides the bee sting I was only ever frightened by creepy-crawlies once. Auntie Vera padded the seat of my red pedal car with newspapers to protect my bony bottom, and during one of my returning visits to my mother and father in town, a hugh hairy huntsman made its home amongst the paper. As soon as I sat in my car again, all set for a sweeping joy-ride around the paths, the huntsman ran from its hiding place, up my side and sat on my shoulder. That hairy monster with glittering beady eyes, its leg span almost as big as my tiny face, was enough to send me into the only fit of hysteria I ever had.

There is one picture which stays vividly in my mind as revelation of how things are, which occurred in my grandparent's bedroom at Buen, which seems to be important to relate. Grandma and Auntie Vera had just fluffed up the mattresses and as I was about to jump into a shaft of sunlight angled right into the room, I noticed something which seemed to be extraordinary. I had been running in and out, disturbing the patch of light on the otherwise darkened bedroom floor. I saw right then before my eyes that the beam of light was not a pure, clear golden shaft, but instead the air revealed in its light was dense with moving particles. I realized that the world around me was always filled with moving life invisible to our normal eye in everyday circumstances.

3. The presage

My second birthday had been an occasion for it was then that my father had presented me with what was to be a treasured possession . . . a doll called Sylvia. She came in a long slim box, the kind that I now associate with the presentation of long-stemmed roses. The box was silver and there on the bottom, at her feet on the outside of the box, was her name written in fine flowing script. She was blonde and blue-eyed, not a baby doll but a delicate little girl who could cry and go to sleep. On my third birthday I was given a china teaset made in Japan. Although I did not know it at the time, on that same day, war was declared in Europe.

The next few months seemed no different at the time. I still continued to spend many happy days out at Buen. Auntie Vera taught me to do simple embroidery and although books and stories did not yet feature strongly on my agenda I learnt what it was to love and care for a household. Grandma and Auntie Vera were skilled in every womanly accomplishment of the time.

My mother was never a true homebody. Rather than make jam, she preferred to sink windmills with 'Dad and Uncle Gordon, or help my father in his bike and electrical shop. Pregnancy was always an illness to her but as soon as Graeme was born in 1940 she opened her milk bar and sweet shop just beside my father's enterprise, hoping, I suppose, that she could carry on a part of the shop when my father enlisted. Graeme spent the first few months of his life almost under Mum's wing in a cot in the hallway. When he crawled, he had the whole hallway blocked off at both ends in which to play and all the society of the shop to keep him amused. No wonder he is the most sociable creature of all our family.

I have little recollection of my mother at that time, except for one vivid picture of her arriving out at Buen to make a ball gown. All day without relief, she sewed that dress. She was a slight, dark-haired young woman at that stage; gay, vivacious, high spirited, irreverent in her humour and obviously very happy and fulfilled. Auntie Vera said that Max and Zena were the picture-book couple: attractive, clever, very much in love and well suited to each other and, until the war came along, seemed to have the world at their feet. That dress was a froth of ice blue and white tulle scattered with groups of silver and blue sequins. I watched with fascination as Auntie Vera painted my mother's shoes with silver frost.

The war first showed its hand when Auntie Vera married a soldier. She left us to spend a short time with Uncle Clive before he went on active duty. Her residence with her new mother-in-law on the other side of Mudgee felt as though she was on the other side of the world rather than seventy miles away. The morning after her wedding, I went searching for my beautiful new purple satin hair-ribbon which had dropped from my head as I was carried, asleep in a blanket, from the sulky the previous night. I found it just outside the front gate, almost all of its colour leached into the earth beneath it by the morning frost. All the feelings of loss and the flood of unspoken fear for the future centred on the spoiled ribbon . . . I was inconsolable. I was right, nothing would be the same again.

Soon my father went off to war. Uncle Gordon followed and even the son of our local "Sir" was not exempt. 'Dad could not get help for the farm so most of it was leased on agistment and he and Grandma moved into town to live with my mother.

My father's cousin Lloyd was a commercial artist and his letters came with small drawings on the envelope which sometimes gave a clue to their whereabouts. Almost every letter had some of it cut by the Forces' censors, but the news most badly missed and which gave us the greatest sense of distance and parting was that lack of knowing where they were. My father was in Darwin at the time of the Japanese air raid and later on leave brought home a photo of it. When he was sent to New Guinea, he seemed already an eternity away.

During one of the letter-reading sessions in the lounge, the death of Ian McMaster, only son of Sir Frederick, was discussed. The possibility of my own father being killed was as remote to me as he was. It was the sort of thing that only happened to other familes. It would not happen to ours.

4. April 7, 1943

The phone in the hall rang twice like a low alert to the most responsible person in the house. My grandmother's voice was low and questioning, and then her words became dispersive and troubled in their tones. Like the sound of indistinct gunfire in the hills, muffled and unpredictable, her words came to me as a picture that was there, powerful in its colour but its clarity blurred and its message incomprehensible.

This day, the seventh of April, 1943, was the most critical day of my life. As the Christian world measures its progress backwards and forwards from the birth of Christ, I measure mine back and forth from that April day.

No one actually told me for some time that my father was dead; that he had been accidentally killed at war. My mother was bundled into my grandmother's bed where she lay not seeing or hearing my cries. I don't think I actually cried out loud, but mothers usually hear that kind anyway. Dr Bray arrived to do something to her and sometime during the morning I was taken to play for the day with the Banbury children. I don't know who walked beside me up the cattle track to the house.

"Where is my Daddy?" I asked.

"He's gone to heaven," the person said.

"Won't he ever come back to live with us?"

"No, he's gone to live with God."

"You mean he won't come back for ever and ever?" I persisted.

"No," came the answer.

I wanted to ask more questions but I didn't know exactly what. It all seemed so unsatisfactory.

"But can't he come back just for a little while? We haven't said goodbye to him, you know." I don't know what my poor companion said to that.

The day was slow and grey: right into my subconscious it was grey. I played all day at the Banburys. They seemed so quiet treating me as though I might break or tear apart in some way. All through those long, long hours of doleful playing, I wanted to go home. Didn't my mother want me home?

I've no idea where my brothers Graeme and Brett went that day or how Pop and Ma King got through that first day of the different world. Everything seemed to have melted into the soft grey nothingness, and I could not even distil its shocking blast into a comfortable silver chain of tears. There were no links with the dead and the living were locked in a chasm of deadened life which follows a catastrophic dislocation of their reality.

In the kitchen her mother sat, her feet in the oven of the wood stove, stitching away the empty minutes. The faint warmth of the room and the repetitive rhythmical movements of her fingers, lulled her senses and salved the open wounds within her. Into the quiet a low keening curled to prize awake her consciousness.

A singing crying came to her, a misty column of crooning sound which rose, hung in the air and then drifted away into the silent night.

The child lay on her side, arms encircling her doll, head and body enclosed in the aspect of protection, rocking imperceptively in the bed in tune with her song of grief. "Stop it," her mother said in a vehement whisper, "you'll wake the boys. Stop upsetting yourself." She shook the child to wakefulness. "And everyone else. Crying won't bring him back. Go to sleep."

The child's eyes flew open, her arms unfurled from her doll and she turned over, her face turned away from her toy. From there she could not see her mother, whose eyes were distraught and whose face was creased with lines of contained despair. The mother patted the child's back until sleep came.

She returned to the kitchen, where she stirred the fire to smouldering, reluctant life.

The watching world of the night stood by. All was still to the eye and the ear of the day, but it only had the stillness, the senselessness of the corpse — the sleepy sound of the night is just a veil, a shade, a side of the reality that has no shape, no voice and no end.

Child's prayer

God bless Mummy and make her better soon. My grandad is very good at nursing me, but I want my

Mummy. God bless Daddy and give him my love. Tell him I miss him so badly that Sylvia and I feel sick in our heads. I wish I knew where heaven was. My mother says it's where all good children go when they die. I just wonder when I'm going to die! Is heaven somewhere near New Guinea, God? I don't understand really because my kitty's gone to heaven and he didn't live near New Guinea — he lived with me.

God bless Brett and Graeme and make them good too. God bless my grandma and grandfather and keep them safe. God bless Pop and Ma and help them not to feel so sad.

My Daddy told me in his last letter to look after Mummy and be a good girl. You know God I do try but we really do need our Daddy. Can't he please come back to us? If I'm a very good girl will you let him come back?

In the early hours of the morning, just before the deepest part of the night which precedes the dawn, my mother crept into the bed beside me. She hardly woke me for her movements were careful. There was no doubt she was spent, exhausted, numb with the cold and loss of feeling.

We lay there, doll and child and lone parent; together in the bed, separated and separate in the way we were affected by our mutual loss. My brothers slept in beds beside us in the room — God knows what dreams they dreamed, but they were too young to make clear connections between events or to make sense of them. We had been a family, encircled by our shared feelings, our envisaged future and the interwoven activities of daily life. Now, one had been taken from us and we felt the loss as a true dismembering. We felt the pain of it as surely as if a limb had been torn from our very own flesh, from our very own bodies!

We became a family again but my mother never recovered from that death. For the last thirty years of her life, the only way she could get the feeling of life and warmth into her being, was to take a daily dose of the spirit drink. I was to discover in adulthood that the pain of the lost part of you has to be experienced eventually. For the time being, my own pain was enough to bear — it was almost overwhelming so that some pain was placed in storage, gathering to tidal wave proportions, waiting its turn to move into my consciousness.

At some time in our lives we learn that we cannot leave the shape of our futures to other people, for that is the gift that only children have a right to. But aged seven, discharged from my father's care and briefly from my mother's warming arms, I was as alone as I would ever feel. Out of that feeling came the first hint of my decision to take charge of myself, and never to rely on anyone else's care for my happiness. I was very young to have that knowledge — my loss of innocence came early and with it, burdens too heavy for my unformed shoulders.

Every day, my father's pet cockatoo had called out to his owner from his hollow tree home in our backyard. "Max, Max, Max," he would shriek whether my father was home or not. On the day that my father was killed, the bird was silent. He never spoke again and within a month, he too was dead.

A dream: The giant appears

On very hot summer days, we would all lie around at Buen like lizards, hoping that our stomachs or a bare patch of skin would contact a cool surface of floor. We would lie there, panting, stupefied by the weight of the heat on our consciousness, blinking, moving in and out of that half world which lies between sleep and waking. On these occasions I wouldn't be sent to my bed in Auntie Vera's room outside on the verandah. I was allowed to share the larger space of the loungeroom where a faint breath of moving air would travel right through the house from the front to the back door — that is, if there was one.

This was the setting of a dream I had three times during my childhood, probably when my father went away, just after he was killed, and later when the new father was in the offing.

I was dressed in a dusty pink headcloth dress which was smocked beautifully, but in quite uncharacteristic colours for either my mother or my aunt. I had always imagined that Auntie Vera had made that dress for me, but Mum assured me it was she who had made it. Who knows!

I was sitting on my haunches, or lying looking at something, playing, directly in line with the front and back doors. This was called the hallway, although it only had one wall and a carpet runner. In the midst of my playing I felt a presence, more oppressive than the heat of the afternoon. In the doorway, blocking the light, stood a giant of a man. I was deeply and instinctively afraid. We had been taught to be wary of visiting strangers to the farm because of the common land nearby, which often housed swaggies and other travellers of unknown origins. My Grandma never turned people away, strangers or not, without offering them food and drink. This stranger was different. To my horror she now offered him afternoon tea. How couldn't she see the danger? How could her goodness blind her to his evil?

His shadow fell across me, truly obliterating my light, and as he came into the room to sit down opposite my grandmother, his eyes held me still. He ate and he drank, keeping me within his gaze. I felt like a toy, drained of my power, waiting for my Master to pick me up, to do with me what he willed.

I managed to come to my self, knowing that no one could save me. I tried to get past him to my room outside on the verandah. His great long legs stretched across the room like the legs of an uncurling spider. As I tried to climb across them, they seemed like hurdles, like mountains, like boulders, like fences, like impossible odds to a frightened, alone little girl fighting for her life. I was indeed fighting for my life for I knew that if the giant got me, he would devour me — eat me up — eat me up as surely as he was eating my grandmother's cakes and tea.

In desperation I made for the door, I tripped, I scrambled, I fell, I got to my knees and I ran.

Inside the bedroom, I slammed the door. I watched the door knob slowly turn beneath my childish grip.

He came. He came in upon me and began to eat me up. In the horror I burst through to a stillness like death. Only my consciousness of Being remained in the world . . . I no longer had my body . . . then I woke up.

How powerful the word is. I have carried this dream within me for close on forty years. I have dreamed it three times, but it is nothing now as I see it before me — out of me — an experience cut from me like a canker. I see its significance now as I see my words.

5. Glimpses of silent fears

The blood of the day was not yet running. All around was anaemic; just tinted with the colour of pearl. People still in their beds were turning over to catch the morning but their pulses were still slow and even from their sleep.

Dressed from head to toe in my winter woollies, I jumped in the puddles in the empty road, shattering their fragile icy covering as if to wake something up. The horse, harnessed and ready to go in the sulky, stamped its feet on the road, and snorted, sending streams of snowy white breath into the steely cold atmosphere. Here and there a chimney was blowing a thin pillar of smoke, straight up into the cloudless sky. I ran into the cut grass near our side door, disturbing its frosty layer, revealing its winter green colour with my footsteps. My tummy was warm with grandmother's porridge but my feet and my fingers in their woolly hand-mitts were numb and almost bloodless with the chilling cold. Spasmodic sounds of dogs and birds rang into the clean crisp air and were carried for miles. Squares of golden light in neighbours' windows grew paler as the first fingers of pale sunshine crept low and long across the earth. My world was waking up, but only just.

All of a sudden Grandad came bustling through the door, arms full of provisions. Grandma followed trailing an extra travelling rug and giving last-minute instructions in her deep warm voice. Before I knew it, I was hoisted into the sulky seat next to 'Dad, rugged round and ready to go. 'Dad gave his whip a brief nimble crack above the horse's ears, then we were off up the cattle track. Up the steep hill we went. When we reached the top of the ridge, our horse Ginger broke into a brisk trot. Here the sunshine was unhindered. Our faces began to tingle as the warmth flowed back into them, blending with the cool air flowing past us.

Great vistas lay on either side of that ridge road. Their solemn silences were punctuated occasionally by carolling magpies, currawongs and crows. Flocks of screeching coloured birds flew across our vision from time to time. Everything seemed to unfold before us in tune with some deep immeasurable rhythm known only to nature. The horse gradually responded to it. We quickened into steep gullies filled with cold and the shadows of hill and bush, sending arcs of silver water out from our wheels as we crossed fords at their depths. Up the other side we dashed, out into the sunlight again. At other times Ginger would stagger up a hill, or walk with deliberate sobriety through shallow creek beds.

These seven miles to the farm filled me with patterns of perception that were to lie within me like a cache of beauty for the rest of my life. I feasted then, as I do now in my memory, on the ribbons of multi-coloured earth exposed in the cuttings — the flesh of mother earth laid bare.

The sound of our passage changed as we turned from the main road into the common which led up to Buen's front gate. Gone was the sharp clip-clop on the corrugations. Here the soil was soft and black on the gently undulating meandering track. Here the bush was deep and untouched — a favourite spot for swaggies to rest in peace and shelter.

As we came out into the open and stopped to unfasten the first of many gates that day, I saw the house. How lonely it looked — left and unloved. It seemed unnaturally silent; no roosters crowed, or dogs barked to mark our arrival. There were no welcoming voices, no smoke or inner lustre to the house that usually expresses the presence of the living. Ginger was released from his labours to graze in the home paddock. We took off our big coats and gloves, then armed with a banana as a special treat, we set off for the bottom paddock where the sheep were to be moved to another paddock. As we walked through the cow yard, swarms of tiny insects rose into the warm air from the dry and disintegrating pads of cow dung. I ran along the sheep track, weaving in and out and behind and in front of 'Dad as we moved like the sheep so many times before, to the lower windmill and the largest water trough on the farm.

"You stay here," said 'Dad already looking up and over the next rise, "the wretched things are not very far away but it might be too far away for you to walk." I jumped on and off large blocks of rock salt watching him disappear over the hill.

Almost at the same instant a deathly quiet descended upon that place. The silence was over-whelming in its intensity but then my ears began to ring and throb with the effort of listening for what could not be heard, nevertheless there was some-thing apprehensible in the atmosphere. Suddenly the air between myself and the hillside seemed alive and potent with menace. It was as if the absence of my grandfather had created a void; it was as if my mere childish presence was not enough to suppress the malevolent forces which had guarded this countryside and the virgin bush since primeval times. Whether adult senses are too blunted to perceive these ancient sentinels, or the civilized strength of a farmer like my grandfather normally sent them into discreet retreat, I do not know, but there and then my child's awareness discerned their presence as surely as if they had materialized before me to warn me off.

My apprehension centred in my ears as sounds. It became almost as loud as the song of cicadas in summer. My eyes searched the hills for 'Dad's return but there was nothing but spreads of winter grass and sheep tracks on the brown slopes, and here and there a tree stump.

My eyes nearly burst from scanning the hillside, moving like a camera looking for the principal character in a vital piece of film. Still he did not come. I strained my ears to hear some evidence of him shouting at the sheep but the ringing silence overcame all.

I began to walk up the hill in an effort to get a view of the other side but my eyes kept returning to a shape-filled blackened tree stump half way up the hill over to my left. 'Dad had taught me to recognize the smell of a fox and I fancied that I could smell one now. Fear flowed through me, smearing my vision and blocking my ears with vibrating surging blood. I knew there were foxes about right now because I had heard Auntie Vera telling Mum that one had been disturbed in a hen house and that it had attacked the farmer's wife when she had found it. There had been drought conditions and rabbits were scarce. There was no telling what a fox might do when it was hungry. After all I was seven, only seven years old and slight for my age. The stump began to move in my vision and the sun's haze shifted its outline until I could bear it no longer — I turned and ran. I probably ran all the way back to the sulky where I felt hot and just a little hungry but not yet safe. My hat came off, I picked up another banana and set off for my home in town — seven miles away.

I remember little of that trip but I do know that once I got on to the much travelled road not one person passed me on the way, and although I was alone I no longer felt in danger. I travelled along recreating the horse's pace in my own childish way. As I got hotter I discarded pieces of clothing leaving them carelessly by the roadside, but carefully filling my pockets with precious finds as I went. I had no further thoughts for the menacing gully and the moving tree stumps. Nor did I keep in my mind's eye my final view of Buen's house; with its back gate tied up and the wistaria-covered walk to the deserted back door. The twisting gnarled old branches had been exposed and grey — there had been no sign of spring leaf. The brief glance I had given that walk had brought to me a picture of ageing entwined limbs of a shelter which is no longer used. Everything had seemed suspended in some kind of living death. Looking back, that was the feeling of those of us who waited for the war to end — our destinies suspended, while waiting for the action which would return our loved ones to us.

When afternoon had well and truly replaced the morning and when I was along the ridge road just outside the town, 'Dad came galloping up to me. Ginger was white with sweat, long clouds of white foam fell from his coat as he stopped, trembling with the effort and my grandfather's distress. 'Dad jumped off his back, picking me up a little roughly in his relief. Up into the saddle again we both went, making off for the town at a more solemn pace. 'Dad had looked everywhere for me, back over the hill in case he had passed me, and with absolute dread he had peered into the well at the windmill. At last he had picked up my trail at the sulky.

Ginger was a half draught so that our movements were not exactly sedate or comfortable, but I felt marvellous tucked between the reins and against 'Dad's chest. I could feel his strong heart-beat and I listened to its echo in Ginger's galloping hooves as we neared home. 'Dad set me down at the top of the cattle track whilst he went back to complete his task with the sheep.

Mum and grandma were astounded to see me

arrive alone; filthy dirty, pockets overloaded with beautiful rubbish and looking dishevelled.

"Where is 'Dad?"

"Where have you been"?

"What's happened?" Their eyes and voices lifted like frightened birds flying heavenward, as they heard my garbled story. As if some kind of action on their part would solve the whole problem, they bundled me into bed surrounding me with fluffed up cushions and a feather eiderdown, feeding me a teaspoon of emergency medicine — warm brandy and sugar. For me the excitement was over. All I wanted was a drink, a biscuit and a play with the kids.

That night I fell asleep on 'Dad's knee by the fire. That day I had imagined fear, seen its manifestations, and had fled from it and arrived home safely. My sleep was as still and untroubled as the valleys around.

Unfortunately it was not always so. My doll Sylvia and I would cry ourselves to sleep after my father went to the war and was killed. I would cuddle her moaning with grief until my mother came — her own well of grief prised open by my own.

Like the good girl I was thought to be I would slip into sleep, where I would be pursued by Japanese soldiers. They would come through locked doors, always from the cattle track where we often saw our own troops moving in trucks by the dozen to camp further north where they trained before serving overseas. The noise was interminable as the line of convoy passing our house, and the dust followed me into sleep, choking my breath into asthmatic seizures and paralysing my limbs in dream as I fled in my little red car to Buen. Up and down the hills I pedalled, forded streams and dry creek beds, changing to an elephant when heavy rains overflowed the creeks. At last at Buen, I would find it empty, and as I walked about the paddocks I would hear the air raid siren and then the planes above my head flying low. I would try to run or even crawl but it was no use. I would wake, my blood slowed to a painful pace in my legs, crying for help.

Someone would rub the life into my legs again and my mother would lather my chest with a mustard plaster to warm my lungs into rhythmical action again.

My pursuers were never German. It was the Japanese who killed my father, and it was the Japanese who followed my pathways in sleep. We heard after my flight from the fox at Buen, that a German prisoner-of-war was caught that day, not far from my course. My family caught their breaths but I was not concerned — my enemies had flat yellow faces with eyes almost closed, and tiny bodies not much bigger than my own. They came in convoys, night after night.

The day that peace was declared in Europe, I heard the news while sitting on our side step, finishing a jumper in the sun. My legs became useless and while the chatter of excitement surrounded me, 'Dad sat me on the kitchen table to massage the strength back into my body again from the feet up. He did a good job, for later I joined the revellers, wearing my Red Cross veil and my good white dress. I marched around the town singing and chanting with joy, and playing games on the oval until nightfall.

At a dinner party recently a middle-aged man declared that my generation was lucky — they knew nothing of war. I reacted sharply, but how could I compare the despairing dream and changed destiny of a young child with the damage done to that man, for he had been trained to kill his brother man. In the years ahead, when life became simpler, when plans could be made again, my fear did not go away — it simply hid away and changed its form.

6. The terrifying tread of a giant recedes

I had my first asthma attack when I was eighteen months old. The attacks grew so severe and so frequent that in my seventh year, my mother took me to Sydney to see a specialist.

During one of the many visits to Prince Alfred I was given six injections in my left arm to ascertain my allergic reaction to common things, such as house dust and bananas.

The injections were not just little pricks in the skin as we have now, but real full size injections. By the sixth both my mother and I had lost our brave front and were crying together. Kapoc, close contact with cats, and dogs, bananas, pepper and dust were deemed no no's.

I was organized to stay at Buen for six months, away from the cattle track dust, and house dust as well. In town I suspect there was no time for scrupulous housework, and little inclination by my mother to do it. Every Saturday for six weeks I had to visit Dr Bray for an injection which would help me to build up an immunity to the allergies. Every visit was a hateful procedure. I would sit terrified, hearing the clattering of glass and steel on the other side of the waiting room door, smelling the pungency of methylated spirits, and finally sitting with my head turned away waiting for the painful stabbing of an unwelcome substance into my thin, small arm.

"You're as thin as a married magpie," Dr Bray would say. That night sitting propped in my grandmother's bed I would watch the dancing light on the walls — the dancing light from the loungeroom fire, shifting the shadows into the corners of the bedroom. I would nurse my swelling, throbbing arm into the soft mound of feather pillows. Memories of mustard plasters filled my mind and I felt again the loving fingers of my mother as she wound the warm poultice across my tightened chest. The plasters gave me short-term relief, but the tender administration that went with them stayed as long as the comfort. In contrast the injections felt like small wounding, but they were to bring me the first long period of freedom to breath easily.

School was suspended for the time being so instead I took correspondence lessons as my mother had done before me. Sometimes Mum and the boys came out to visit, but most of the time I was alone. When they were gone I would look out of the window imagining they were still there, hearing my mother's voice saying, "Now, when you are wheezy

43

you must not run about outside in the cold. You'll get too excited and get yourself sick again."

When the wheezes really did start in earnest, I had a new magic puffer with Expaxadrene which would give me immediate relief, unless it was a massive attack. Previously nothing had helped and when I first had felt my breathing begin to restrict and my lungs to contract, I would often question my mother earnestly, "Mummy am I getting truly, really sick again?" She told me later, that these words would almost make her cry because at that time there had been little that could be done.

As the wheezing had increased and the breathing became more laborious and exhausted, my mother had been filled with dread. All she had been able to do was give me those mustard plasters as hot as my heaving chest could bear. She would hold me loosely on her lap where her own warmth and rhythmical breathing could still my fear and help to keep up my ebbing strength.

When I returned to school and home things were different. I had to repeat a grade for the things I had learnt on the farm were not the skills of the schoolroom. The district inspector arrived and decided this. He asked me to read to the class a story from the reader which I had never seen before. I was not yet accepted by my classmates. In my absence they had re-formed their friendship groups. I looked and sounded different from everyone I had spent the first year with. I was pale, thin, hiding in my body, quiet in voice, nervous and shy. Standing there in front of them all, beginning again as a stranger I failed the test and felt a failure.

In the playground I was taunted, "Skinny King,

Skinny King." In an orgasm of spite I was spaced inside a column of rubber tyres which grew taller and taller as the children heaped one upon the other, until this stack was feet above my head. The light came to me from above and the voices chanting, "Skinny King, Skinny King" were muffled and far away. I don't know how it all ended but after that I gradually became one of them again.

At about this time my mother was taken to Mudgee Hospital to have her appendix removed. Grandma and 'Dad came to town again to look after us, but to be without my mother was terrible. She was of course, after our father's death, the centre of our lives.

One morning, so that I felt that I had some control over my life, although it was not a conscious thought, I insisted on wearing my best dress to school. It was a white Red Cross dress, but as it was not a Red Cross Day my grandparents refused to let me wear it. I cried myself into a fit of despair. My grandfather took me, unable to stop crying, to school. Inside the gate my vehement conversation was interpreted by the school teacher's daughter as swearing. I was sent inside to think about my behaviour and await my punishment. That morning we had heard from the hospital that my mother would have to remain there for another week and when Mr Caines, the teacher, came to sort out my almost hysterical weeping, I managed to tell him that I thought my mother was going to die. The crying and the unusual sympathy it evinced from Mr Caines brought me back to myself and into a period of relative quiet and normality.

Mr Caines had always taught by fear — physical

and mental intimidation. Some people fluff up their feathers to perform at their peak in those conditions, but I believe in the power of love, co-operation, trust; in the ability of people to perform their best from within themselves. A bully gives you no room to give the best of yourself. When he stood there, stern and crew-cutted, he would bark, "Seven and eight?" Instead of fluffing up I would withdraw, performing only from my mechanical memory, uninvolved in the learning, but deeply assaulted in my being. Nevertheless in the following year, I topped the class and whispered the answers too difficult to Judy Orth, my best friend who sat next to me and was in the class above me now. Mr Caines came grudgingly to respect my art work, and in the eyes of the other children I had special talent. When I drew I became as one with everything and oblivious of the everyday world. I worked swiftly, in complete harmony with myself, bringing to life on paper what I had seen, loved and thought significant. The knowledge that light transformed a leaf into a capsule of colours while giving an illusion of green to us, lived in my fingers as I drew. Sometimes I was surprised at the pictures I created. Had I really drawn them? Where had they come from if I had not?

I have often wondered at Mr Caines' uncharacteristic kindness to me on that upsetting day of my mother's relapse. His cruelty was not in my imagination, for as soon as young men became available as teachers again, he was dismissed. I suspect that on that one occasion he had demonstrated a sneaking regard for my mother, for although she did not fit the role of submissive woman which he usually admired — she was forthright and a fighter — those qualities would catch his respect. He could never have understood my wish to wear my nurse's uniform to school to assist my mother's healing. He could not identify with my unconscious act but he could understand my mother's battle, in this case through me. Our mother was fiercely protective where our welfare was concerned. Many people had offered to adopt each one of us but she would not entertain the thought. Even when a wealthy and sophisticated great-aunt arrived from Sydney, sporting some of the finery from her smart Manly millinery shop, and offered to take me back to enrol me in a girls' school to make me into a little lady, my mother was not impressed. The sight of me playing football with the boys in the paddock over the road, skirting in and out of the cow pats, shouting and getting as dirty as the boys, prompted Auntie Zita to propose the idea. My mother preferred to leave me in my play, thankful for the regained health that made such play possible and for the very obvious tie of family that held us so closely together. We had indeed become a very close family, the four of us.

One summer holiday I grabbed a box of matches from the Buen pantry, gathered up Graeme and Brett as enforced voluntary labour to set fire to the short grass in the home paddock. As each tussock of tinder dry grass caught alight, so did my imagination. The whole force, the consuming energy of fire seemed to take hold of me. I frantically lit more, urging the boys to hurry their endeavours so that all the tussocks would be alight at the same time. What a show it would make! What a mighty force we would have engaged. I had no thought for the consequences — I was only intent on my service to the fire. Somehow almost wishing to become all consuming, all transforming, all powerful.

Thank goodness someone in the house smelt the evidence of our mischief. Their noses were of course tuned to the smell of fire at that time of year. Soon a bucket brigade had doused the fire in its journey towards the next-door paddock. There Sir Frederick McMaster's lush chest-high hay waited to be harvested.

When the fire was quenched, we three were lined up outside the bathroom, waiting for a good hiding with Grandad's razor strop — administered by our mother. I was last so that I had longer to wait and think about my irresponsible behaviour. Poor Mum, she was always very fair and our warnings were very clear. But in the matter of safety she had to be hard. We never thought of her actions as cruel. Thank goodness, on this occasion, Grandad came in from the paddocks just as I was getting my first stinging belt. He rescued me, saying "Zena, you're too hard on that little girl." That little girl collapsed in relieved weeping into her grandad's strong arms.

As we grew older we were given bikes and then our world increased in miles of travel and adventure. For hours we could be without adults to check how clean our faces, our knees, or our hands were, to check whether our hair was done, or suggest that we should put on a coat or take one off. Out in the countryside we were just ourselves with no one to answer to but nature itself. Pure air, warming sunshine, cleansing rain, breaking up frost and the utterly predictable change of season to season.

What more could I have wanted? The war had ended and by the time a few years had passed, I became confident of my good health. Trips to hospital with asthma or congestion of the lungs became incidents of the past rather than constant possibilities. But there was something which we children felt we needed. Other children, every child we knew at that time, had a dad. It was the *idea* that appealed to us rather than the actuality of having someone to fulfil the role in everyday life. By 1948 when such a thing became a possibility our mother and we three children had become a self-sufficient happy unit. Many suitors dipped their hats at our mother, but no one was given special favour.

On the surface Mum resumed her bright and lively way of speaking and relating to others. She was tiny, a half inch over five foot tall, and slight. Her hair was very dark and softly curled. As she told a story (she was a good raconteur) or glided around the dance floor in the local hall, she would be alive with the immediate enjoyment of it all. On Anzac Day though, and on anniversaries of our father's death, her face would take on the countenance of a person haunted. Her eyes then looked into another world. They would fill with shadow and her skin would lose the warm tinge of freely running blood. Once again, on these days, she would be lost to me.

Her suitors knew how to please my mother — they would arrive with chocolates or lollies for us, the children. Sweets were rare fare for us so that the enjoyment we felt was quite evident and made its mark on our mother. A gentle-voiced bee farmer was my favourite. I didn't like the other, a coarse-featured shearer with dangly curls and wide flaring trousers. I didn't like the new baker either, even though one day in the shop he made me a gingerbread man. He had a sense of humour I did not understand and there was something about him I did not trust. It wasn't a romantic interest my mother and her friend Alma showed him. Soon after he arrived the two women noticed that he was never without his hat. He wore it everywhere — in the shop, while he was baking, and even at the dinner table. Mum and Alma were intrigued and devised a plan which should have revealed the secret beneath the hat. Eeling was a favourite pastime for all families and newcomers were often introduced to it as a local treat, peculiar to our village life. The plan was to take the baker eeling and in the hubbub of Alma thinking she had an eel on her line, Mum would pretend to fall into the creek. When the baker would attempt to save her Mum would knock off his hat in a wild flurry of hands and arms. The trouble was that the baker's loyalty was not as the women predicted. On the edge of the creek, at about three o'clock on a chilly morning the baker held on to his hat, leaving my mother to fall screaming with indignation into the unwelcoming water, taking Alma with her.

"You're only trying to knock off my hat . . . you bloody wretches," yelled the baker, stomping off home without a gentlemanly glance at the guilty culprits in the creek.

They discovered later, that all the poor man was trying to do was to hide a prematurely and completely bald head, the result of some unusual disease.

There was another experience that ended in disaster too, and caused as much amusement for my mother. This was of a different kind. A fellow from Coolah was courting both my Mum and a woman who worked in the Coolah Post Office. The silly fellow wrote to them both, but in his excitement perhaps, placed the wrong letters in the already addressed envelopes. My mother thought it a great joke, but the woman from Coolah decided to make the man choose and he did eventually marry her.

7. An introduction

One afternoon in the shop, now used for Mum's dressmaking, I was introduced to a dapper little man, dressed immaculately in a green sports coat and grey flannels. He had the cleanest shoes I had ever seen apart from the legendary shine of Ma King's brother, Horace's. He had a small, kind round face which was open, smiling and generous. His beautiful hat was handled with the air of a gallant but I could see that his wish to please was quite genuine and not just part of the manners he had obviously acquired.

For the length of the shearing season, stretching from late August to mid-December, "Roy the Boy" as this man was called in the sheds, and his mate "Reckless Dan" were to be seen at every local entertainment. Those men worked extremely hard in very poor conditions so when the working week came to a close, they played as hard as they had worked. Roy Mott was the gun shearer and in some ways an exception to the shearing breed. He was well known for his skill and for his reliability. Shearers in early days were not always known for being reliable; the unpredictability of their life, such as the unknown length of time of each shed, the weather and its consequences, the conditions of work and the nature of the team which changed each time it re-formed, probably contributed to the need for a flexible attitude to whatever came along. I suppose, too much flexibility as a result of things beyond your control can drain a person's sense of his own responsibility. I was to learn that this did not apply to Roy Mott.

According to the rules and attitudes of his mates he was a white man, a true blue, a mate to be trusted and admired. In particular cases, these men were fair in their treatment of any man, black, white or brindle. An individual Aborigine working next to them on the board was simply one of the boys, but boongs in general were considered outside their society. Not only were they racist, in general they had no respect for men who did not work with the sweat of their own labour. Men who inherited wealth were despised, and men who worked with their heads had no brains — that is, they had no common-sense. Someone would remark, "They couldn't fight their way out of a paper bag." As for women — they were God's gift to men and therefore to be treated with love and respect. They were to be protected from the hurly-burly of life; they were to stay at home, displaying their gentle womanly arts and that meant being feminine. Women's voices were to be soft, gentle, compliant and thankful to the men who went out into the world to "slave their guts out" to bring home a decent living wage.

All this I was to come across, epitomized in Mr Mott; all these ideas I was to fight against yet still respect the man who introduced these attitudes to me. I was in fact destined to love this man as a father, not by title or by virtue of tie of blood, but because of his deeds — he did, by his own hands and the acts of his heart, become a true father to me. I was to learn that we do not need to take on or even admit the values of another person to be able to meet them in mutual respect, but that was still a very long way off.

Twice I had heard my mother proposed to — once through the loungeroom keyhole, and once while I was quietly doing the beans in the sleepout. While one of the swains was trying to plight his troth in the middle of my Mum's preparation of the Sunday roast! When she finally did accept Roy's, I was not there.

One night I woke to the low thrum of a radio, an alien sound in that late spring night. Its crackles of static were punctuated by erratic gales of sound, rising like waves almost to drown the excited voice of the commentator. I could not hear a word but the quality of the sound was unmistakable. Thoughts of tribal warfare and male confrontation now prick at my consciousness as I recall my feelings at that time. Once I had truly heard what lay behind the single words of the noise, I could not sleep.

Did I call out or did my mother simply make a routine check on her brood? She appeared next to the bed, shading a small torch-light with her cupped hand, saying in a whisper, "Are you all right?"

"Yes," I said "but I can't sleep. What's that terrible noise Mummy?"

"Mmmm," she said, "Mr Mott and I are listening to a world title fight . . . " And she added as if my querying silence required further explanation . . . "It's boxing."

"Boxing," I said in wonder. No one in my memory had ever listened to boxing or had ever talked about it.

"Yes. Now go back to sleep."

It was useless. The volume of the sound was decreased when my mother returned to the lounge, but the intensity of the atmosphere rose. The memory related to feeling disturbed me dreadfully. "Kill him, kill him" seemed to live in the rising cries of the crowd carried by the radio. I listened and waited and so a feeling of frustration joined the tension which rose and fell on my stomach like a fist clasping and unclasping.

I lay there in a turmoil, not knowing how to deal with my tumbling emotions, and not recognizing what they truly were.

My mother returned. "Still awake?"

"See," implicating tones, "have a look at this — I don't dare tell anyone yet — it's still a secret. Have a look at my engagement ring."

The flashlight winked into a dark blue stone set in silver on my mother's left hand. I did not know what to say. This was a new experience for me. What does one say when your mother becomes engaged to someone you do not know — someone who was a foreigner.

"Do you like it? Don't you think it's beautiful?" my mother asked.

"Yes," was all I could think to say.

"Now go to sleep this time," my mother said, turning off the torch and tucking me up for what remained of the night.

I curled up like a hedgehog, a small disquieted and bemused child, feeling the cold and empty space in the bed beside me, usually filled by my mother's warm back. Some time during that vital exchange between my mother and myself the fight had reached its peak — blood had been spilt and now all was quiet.

The fight was truly over. One man had been vanquished and my mother had come to announce the winner of the other battle which had been played out at the same time. Even though my mother was replacing my dear father in her life, my emotional secret self refused to acknowledge my father's death in this way — in fact all announcements of his death were to that part of me a terrible mistake. Within that secret self, I nursed the fantastic illusion that one day he would return home as alive as ever, after years of being secreted away as if in a sacred trust, by some esoteric New Guinea tribe. From time to time I would take this picture out of its hiding place to examine it before putting it away again. It was not to be lost or given up until as a young woman in my late teens I fell in love for the first time. This first experience of love between man and woman was uncomplicated and served to fill the yearning I had had for the unreserved, uncritical and unqualified kind of love I had so briefly experienced with my own father.

Back in my mother's bed on that well-remembered night, my heart and my head overflowed with confusion and I longed for the blankness of sleep. "Our Father which art in Heaven". . . I murmured. I prayed that the angels would come to carry me off, to soothe me and to mend the wound my mother could not see.

The chant of the sacred pledge and the sensing towards something beyond myself gathered me up as if I were in the arms of the true Father. Now sleep came quickly; soon I had joined my brothers in the rest of unconsciousness.

On the December 30, 1948, my mother and Roy Mott were married in Mudgee. Without thinking, we three children had bundled ourselves into the bridal car with the newly married pair, as they prepared to drive away from the church. There was much laughter and a little consternation, but Father, as we now called him, welcomed us saying that we were a new family together and that we may as well begin as one.

The decision to call him Father was not an easy choice. Daddy, Pop and Dad had already been taken. Father seemed a little formal, but somehow it was right at that stage; it designated the role he was undertaking rather than his personhood.

I enjoyed the wedding preparations — its sense of occasion, my mother's beautiful new clothes, and most of all feeling very important as I took the boys to buy our wedding present. We were given seven pounds and despatched to the biggest store in Mudgee to buy something suitable. Brett and Graeme trailed along behind me, a little bored. I resolutely steered them to the crockery and glass-ware section. There on a glass shelf, reflected in a mirror-backed wall, I saw just the thing — a large jug which could be an ornament, or a receptacle for flowers. The thing that had caught my eye was its colours.

Mum and Father spent the next few weeks travelling all over New South Wales meeting various relatives to establish the new order. I don't know where the boys went, but I spent those summer holidays with my grandparents, Uncle Gordon, Auntie Rene and their young baby.

At first it was strange to be with my grandparents away from the farm, but I spent many happy times with 'Dad. He would dink me on his bike, carpentry tools strapped in a bag to the bar, to the site of one of the houses he was building. With the amount of skill and industry 'Dad expressed, he should have been a rich man, but he rented these houses to families at rates he thought they could afford. One house was occupied by a widow for years for almost no rent at all. My grandparents lived as simply as they had always done on the farm. Most afternoons I spent sweeping, hammering, holding implements for 'Dad, but in the morning I hovered about Grandma as she bottled or preserved fruit, or I followed Auntie Rene while she bathed baby Gavin. Auntie Rene had waited some time for Gavin's arrival. In her fortieth year her baby was so precious to her that she created around her an atmosphere of intense love — she seemed to savour every task associated with that baby.

At the end of the holidays, Father had to go crutching to the far north while Mum went to Moama to find a new house for us. By late January she had packed up our Cassillis home and on a brilliant sunny morning in early February, my mother, the boys and I raced about the streets saying last minute goodbyes. Ma King in tears, watched as we piled into the removal van beside the driver. As he turned to drive over the bridge and out of Cassillis, Ma King's white handkerchief waving to us was the last thing I saw. It took three days to travel what was two thirds of the distance of New South Wales. From the elevated view of the ranges we gradually descended, and on the last day and night of our journey we saw nothing but open, flat land. At the time we were filled with excitement and captivated by the newness, but as I look back, I see that journey as an uprooting, an awful transplanation. It took three days to get to a place that was as foreign as another country, and a life that was to anneal me in a way yet unforeseen. The days of my protected, all-loving childhood were over. The ingenuous child who saw beauty in the kingfisher jug, was left behind in the soil of the mountains.

8. Adolescence

A great weight of water gouges a path, meandering from mountain through plains, making a natural division between states, until it finally reaches the sea. Our new home was still in New South Wales, but only just. At thirteen, I stood on the edge of the Murray River bank, at the bottom of our backyard, watching the water flow past. It was as large as a great city highway. On the edges I studied the eddying whirlpools of water as they moved in and around the giant roots of the overhanging gums. This river was awe-inspiring. It was dark and strong and who-knew-what-else, in its depths. How different from the shallow, clear, sparkling water that had run over the stones at Cassillis. This was a river to get to know; this was a river to respect. Every time a paddle steamer came swishing down the river past our backyard, we would tear to the river's edge, watching the enormous red gum logs bobbing in the water behind the frothing, rippling waves, which eventually reached us on the bank.

Everything seemed new. In the street where we now lived, a half dozen families struggled with poverty and hardship. As Father recently remarked, if we'd all pooled our money, it wouldn't have filled a bucket. For the first time, I saw children with bedbug bites and constant impetigo. With a child's natural acceptance of what people are, I saw the essential nature of those half dozen families. They demonstrated their loyalty to each other, accepted us into their neighbourhood with a warmth and enthusiasm. My contact with these simple people whom I learnt to respect was very good training for the work I was to do later in life.

To our sheltered eyes, the lives of these drovers, carriers, strappers and labourers were full of dramatic event. Every Thursday night, I would hear Old Tom, as he was called, riding home on his horse, drunk and full of swearing. I would wake and feel suddenly afraid, not of Tom himself, but of the condition of his life. In the early hours of one morning after a night of illicit drinking, Tom fell from his boat as he rowed home across the river. It was weeks before they found his body. His once powerful body, engorged in life by his drinking, was decimated by the river crays.

One afternoon, while we were exploring the river-bank on our bikes, we discovered a small shack where an old aboriginal woman lived. It looked like a drawing of a child, a one-roomed cottage with miniature garden set out in front, a straight little path flanked with geraniums and small flowers. I was entranced by the unlikely blending of childhood symbol of home and the Australianized version of British country cottage. I paused, looking and thinking, and marvelling at the earth swept so clean, it was as hard as cement. Just then, the old woman appeared through the door, swishing a broom in front of her, sending a hen and chickens scurrying off into the bush to forage for food. Her white hair seemed to gleam in the sunshine in stark contrast to her very dark skin. In the following year, her granddaughter, Esther, was to marry one of Father's shearers. Esther's father was English, and Splinter, as they called her husband, had an Indian and aboriginal parent. He was a very striking man. His dark skin and lustrous, almost black eyes, highlighted a set of beautifully formed gleaming white teeth. Esther shared the bungalow in our backyard with me for the two months before their marriage. It didn't seem at all strange that she, who had barely learnt to read and write, should hear my French verbs in preparation for high school exams.

For the first time in my life, I went to school without fear. I played in the school band, led a team in the school sports, modelled a papier mâché puppet and took part in the writing and performance of the play. Grammar and maths became solid skills instead of intermittent skirmishes. To miss a day of school was an infringement I could hardly bear. The excitement of new subjects such as French and singing in the choir and of new sports was outflanked by my absolute joy in the best teacher I ever experienced. For the first few years, she brought to me regions of knowledge of art and depths of perception that no one else seemed able to do. Every brush stroke of tinted colour was lovingly painted on the Egyptian friezes, which decorated my history of art book. My eyes, so accustomed to the loping, rolling vistas of hills and valleys, now saw the plains and understood the changes in atmosphere and colour that come and go in such an airy vista. The world about me seemed to live in my vision. It was a well of perception from which I drew as I painted.

When Miss Anderson left the school this stream of adventure almost ran dry. I felt cheated as my art experience became meagre and trivial — mere sloshings of paint, of experimenting with nothing but technique. What had been for me a rich vibrant opening of communication became a dead-end mishmash of unrelated wastings of time.

During Forms 1 and 2, I made friends with a girl who had lost her father at the war. We shared secrets, dreams and discovery of changes in our adolescent bodies. We both bought bras long before we needed to. One afternoon, while getting ready for football, I viewed my "yard of pump water" figure with such disgust, I decided to stuff each cup with a sock. This sudden blossoming of body caused short-lived surprise to my girl-friends.

Mel and I spent many hours together at each other's homes. We laughed till our ribs objected, cried in maudlin experimentation, wrote poetry and sketched and painted for hours along the riverbank. Mel was a very strong swimmer and I tagged along as best I could, developing my swimming strength as each long swimming season came by. From September to March, flood waters permitting, we would set off in the early morning on our bikes; spending hour after hour, diving, swimming, and generally revelling in the river. When hunger gripped us, we pedalled furiously home, ate quickly and were eager to be back at the river as soon as parents allowed.

During one of these early summers, three tragedies came to scar the easy landscape of my new emotional life. The first was impersonal, but nevertheless, quite shocking. During a family quarrel between an Aboriginal and his brother-in-law, one was impaled against a wall with a Japanese sword.

The other two deaths were very close indeed. A school friend, Judy, with whom Mel and I had spent hours swimming, contracted encephalitis and died within a fortnight. I was struck again by the suddeness of this terrible disease. One week, looking golden and glistening with the water of our marvellous river, brown-eyed and brown-haired, full of life, and the next, never to be seen again. In a desperate need to escape from the reality of this death, Mel and I sat in the back of the church at the funeral service, whispering of other things, ignoring the real reason for us being there.

One afternoon, when I came home from school, Mum broke the news to me that little Gavin, Auntie Rene and Uncle Gordon's only child, was in hospital, unconscious, also with encephalitis. When he died, I was distraught. I cried through the night, dozing and waking to clutch the only photograph I had of him. The next day at school, I spent half the time fleeing to the toilets, sobbing uncontrollably. I cried for the loss of my little cousin whom I had loved so much during that summer, when my mother had been married. I cried for the cruelty of life.

About this time, I began to be afraid after long periods of quiet happiness, suspecting that the balance was about to be reviewed — that the phantom of death and the possibility of calamitous events was lurking, waiting to overtake me, fracturing my equanimity once more. Dreams of war, and the dream of the giant came back for a time, but then gradually life's blood assumed its normal flow again.

In the autumn of 1951, Mum announced that she

was expecting a child. At first I felt ashamed at such goings on. Mum was old to my eyes; fancy having a baby at her age. But the joy and excitement expressed by my teenage friends, gradually made me realize that it was something to be looked forward to, a perfectly natural event. My mother suffered awful morning sickness right throughout the pregnancy and there were many days when she was unable to do normal housework. I learnt to cook the evening meal during this time and managed to look after the family when she finally went to hospital. On our way home from school we passed Father, who stopped and poked his head through the window of his utility. He looked absolutely green and very excited. "Your mother's gone to the hospital and the baby will arrive at any time".

Cheryl was born that evening, six weeks premature, and when I went to visit Mum the following day in hospital, I imagined she looked as beautiful and peaceful as she had many years previously. She had a soft and tender glow about her. I just loved that little baby and when she was home, I helped to oil her each day until she was old enough to have a proper bath. She'd been an unexpected addition to our family, but once here, she was fêted and fought over. When she was old enough to be pushed in a pram, the three of us guarded over who was going to take her to the baker's shop for the day's fresh bread. She came with us on the wildest escapades, in her stroller or in her pram, and if my mother had known some of the hazards which ranged about her head, she couldn't have failed to believe in a guardian angel. At the beginning of that year, Mum and Father had built their first new home together, closer to the centre of town, and as soon as Cheryl was toddling, Mum began sewing again in an effort to supplement the family income. Esther also had a child and while she helped Mum with hand sewing and general housework, Cheryl and Philip played together in the backyard, oblivious of their naked bodies, so black and so white. I was fascinated. Esther nicknamed Philip "my little black prince". I was a kind of second mother to Cheryl and later, as my mother's health deteriorated, Cheryl and I became close friends as well as sisters.

The year I turned fifteen, I grew five inches and overnight, my legs looked as though they might turn into those of a slender young woman. I became interested in pretty petticoats and planned a grown up wardrobe with smart accessories. Mum took me to buy my first pair of high heels which I thought looked very fetching with their peaked toes. Woe upon woe, after their first wearing, Cheryl's new puppy chewed a great hole in one of the heels, so that was the end of them.

I had the usual number of innocent flirtations with boys of my own age, those kind of hand holding, sly glances in the sixpenny seats at the Friday night picture show, but in my intermediate year, I began going out with a boy I had secretly "fallen for" years previously. Ian was one of those beautiful brown people. His whole being seemed infused with the effects of the summer sun all the year round. His girl-friend before me, by reputation was "fast", and I determined to redeem him. Instead he awakened within me responses I didn't dream existed. It was a time of tender experimentation and sometimes it was disastrous. Thankfully, in the area of this first romance, there was little harm done, only an occasional wrestling with a conscience trying to find ways of expressing love within the bounds of what I came to think of as stupid convention.

I began to wonder why there was one rule for boys and one for girls. It made no sense and seemed to exacerbate the stupid notion that women were either virgins or harlots if they weren't busy being mothers. Why couldn't there be equal relationship, equal initiative, with love running freely from one to the other? The established Church, too, seemed ungenerous in its attitudes. When I invited a Catholic to play in our Church of England table tennis team, a minor storm broke over our church club. The pastor pointed out that if he wanted to play table tennis, he could very well play in his own church team. I thought I'd acted in a Christian way and the pastor's sectarian attitude disappointed me greatly. He had enlivened our church and made it much more relevant to everyday living, but this made it impossible for me to continue in the Church. From my day of confirmation the communion service had always meant a great deal to me. I had actually felt as though the communion enabled me to awaken to spiritual forces and so from time to time, I revisited churches to take communion. Nevertheless, most services seemed to me to be so heavily accented towards sin and death. What I was searching for was enrichment of life and the expression of love. When you are seventeen, death and resurrection seem unimportant.

I was trying all the badges of adulthood and sometimes finding my efforts inappropriate and even dangerous. One weekend, in an effort to be thought grown-up, glamorous, for the obligatory Saturday night dance, I gave my hair a golden blonde rinse. Unfortunately, I became interested in something else during the operation and finished up with bright orange hair gleaming with green lights. I washed and washed it to little avail. I was reluctant to go to school on Monday morning and so I was late. I had the ignominious experience of walking to my place in line in full view of the Monday morning school assembly. One evening I experimented with smoking in our family loungeroom. A car full of young men from the tennis club arrived, taking my attention from the cigarette I had in an ashtray on the armchair. Sitting talking in the car in our drive, we were amazed to see a flickering light on the loungeroom blinds. The local chief of the fire brigade lived next door and thankfully, the couch was doused in professional manner. My mother was furious and her temper not at all appeased, when Ian rang later, gleefully asking if we needed more help from the fire brigade. I was placed under house arrest for six weeks for that misdemeanour.

My last two years at school were filled with sensitive, idealistic searching for the grander meaning of existence in art and literature, and the mechanical, boring process of learning to pass examinations. Through a complicated set of circumstances, and I knew from past experience, certainly not from lack of ability, I failed first go to pass the required number of subjects to qualify for secondary art and craft teacher training. This turned out to be a fortuitous change in direction for, in the light of events in later life breadth of experience was invaluable.

9. No wedding dress for me, please

Teachers' college was for me like a large city of new directions. I revelled in my introduction to psychology, the Greek philosophers, Theban plays, and I enjoyed the practical part of our training. My very first lesson in a class was an art lesson. I felt quite at ease and very happy. My class teacher was a little taken aback by my lack of nerves and warned me against being over-confident. I enjoyed everything about those first two years, the social growing up as well as the basis of academic study.

My first love and I were to be engaged at the end of teachers' college and to be married a year later, but I became caught up with the invitation of a whole world of new experiences. I had a picture of my being shackled to the kitchen sink within those four walls, with an occasional sortie pushing a pram in the streets of the small town in which we lived. I couldn't bear it. It wasn't simply the study or the life experience that I was seeking, it was a conscious wish to develop what was within me to the fullest and also to explore relationships so that I could have a deep understanding of human response. At the end of my two years' training, I was advised to do a third year of art and craft training. Excepting for art history, it all seemed to be very materialistic: experimental, but materialistic none the less. By this time I was really on my own, a young woman with a career and a job to do. I went to the country to teach.

The small village of Balmoral was something I was used to. I played basketball, tennis, swam. I did posters for all the various on-coming village events. I trained a deb set, and drawing on my experience from teachers' college, in company with several others, we put on revues. For the first year in the classroom, I found it very difficult. Art had not been seen as an important subject and the materials I had at my disposal were very meagre. In the cupboard only two feet from the front desks, all I could find was a box of charcoal, a few old boxes of pastels and a fair amount of paper. Somehow I managed, making lots of mistakes and discovering during that time what it was that the children really needed. I'd come to teaching with a very clear idea of what I thought they should have, but of course these two things didn't always go together. On the first day of my second year, I felt as if I was a new person. I had an art room for the secondary students and I'd been able to order the materials myself. From then on we blossomed. The children were a constant source of delight to me and every day over afternoon tea in the teachers' flats with three other young teachers, we shared the charming, incredible and wise things that children had said or done during the day.

I discovered the enjoyment that a group can foster. A half dozen of us, young teachers and local residents, travelled all over the countryside seeking our pleasure. We thought nothing of travelling fifty miles to play tennis, thirty miles to the drive-in and fifty miles home. Sometimes we would tear out of school on Friday afternoon and head for the city to gorge ourselves with city culture and shopping. Back to the country we would come, singing and dancing, inspired by "Salad Days" or "Free as Air" with fresh ideas for our next revue and bursting with enthusiasm for life. It was, for us, a time of salad days and being free as air.

During the second of my three-year stay, I began a relationship with Neil, a young stock and station agent. I am thankful we didn't marry, for although we had our vitality, our love of life and our optimism in common, our values were very different. He had a background of public school life and I found the snobbish ways of some of his friends very hard to take. The practice of judging people by their background, by their clothes, education, or their speech, not only irritated me but filled me with a sense of unfairness. My stepfather had really taught me to see that it is by people's reactions, responses and their innermost thoughts that we should meet others.

During the first weeks of the 1961 school year, I was invited to join the staff of Geelong Teachers' College, as an assistant lecturer in art and craft, taking responsibility for needlework. I thought that I was too young and too inexperienced to take up such a situation. The two senior men were horrified at my answer — to say no to secondment was some kind of heresy. They persuaded me to ring the Department and ask for twenty-four hours to reconsider. That evening I rang the District Inspector, hoping that he might assist me in a realistic assessment of my ability. I discovered that he had recommended my appointment. By the following morning my sense of inadequacy was shot through with sneaking feelings of challenge, and already a few ideas for innovation. I rang the Department and said yes. I knew this was a momentous decision for me, that was to change the course of my life in a way that no other decision had previously. I was turning my back on a simple, perhaps more emotionally satisfying, life. To say yes to the appointment meant saying definitely no to any thought of working through my relationship with Neil. To me, being utterly feminine in the stereotyped way was simply being dishonest. I wanted to develop every attribute I had to the full and to find the best way of expressing it. Going to Geelong was to give me that opportunity. It was difficult to say goodbye to a place which had been so like my early childhood. I'd rested in the love and respect of everyone I knew but what I was about to do would require much more from me.

After the first year of settling in, of finding my feet, of going without a great deal in order to save money, I bought my first car. With wheels beneath me, I was truly independent. What brave but vain strivings. It seemed as though I had an unconscious need to prove my worth or the worth of my life to some unseen judge. Somehow the events of my early life, the calamitous events, prevented me from having a sense of ease about my future. It was as if I felt I needed to make sure things were right, for I could not trust my life to run smoothly or in the way it was meant, without my interference. I was not a competitive person, but I wished to surpass every achievement of my own. Existence seemed to me to be an ever-changing, ever-moving, overflowing globe of filaments of light — each filament a pathway of knowledge, of wisdom, consciousness and of exploring love. Every pathway lured me on to blossom enthusiastically into new growth. Like the fruit trees at Buen, I was to learn that sometimes a cutting back is necessary for a renewal and fructification of life.

10. The sun too has a shadow

There was a ringing roar of sound. It was not just inside me: it spiralled up, up from somewhere deep inside me, engulfing me so that I became that sound and until there was nothing else but that sound — a dinning, spinning, careering crescendo. At the very peak of tumult, before a thousandth of a second could pass, it ceased. I was back, I was conscious. I had been gathered up in that catapulting formation of sound, then hurtled in an explosive effort, through the barrier of consciousness. I was back to earth.

"What in the hell have I done now?" Nothing remained of the all-encompassing noise which had accompanied my breakthrough but a faint far-off tinging in my ears and the gentle swishing to and fro of the windscreen wipers.

"Someone else can turn off my windscreen wipers," I thought. "I'm just too tired."

I seemed to be wrapped in a comforting blanket of inertia — it was a kind of shock absorber, so that the world outside my little car seemed only to exist somewhere beyond me — I could feel nothing. The only stream of life seemed to come to me through my ears; sound was my lifeline.

"I've had an accident," I mused. "And I am only two hundred yards from my destination . . . I can just remember driving up the last hill . . . then nothing!"

A voice, breathy with concern and Saturday night drinking, came to the car window.

"You'll be all right, girlie. Don't move, the ambulance will soon be here."

Move, he says! He must be mad.

Although I had no sense of it at the time, I discovered later that I was lying towards the back with my legs between the front bucket seats.

Tentative sounds floated to me, disembodied voices seemed overcome with the moment, as if in the presence of something they could not understand.

"The young fellow is OK . . . a bit dazed, but walking around."

"The girl is pretty bad," another contributed.

That must be me, I suppose. Oh well, Jess, my friend, I won't be staying with you tonight. You'll have to face marauders alone.

I fell back into my inner world, not even my ears opened their pathway to the outside. I seemed even to be unconscious of my breathing. Slowly, numbed and creeping pain spread over my body until at last, thank God, the ambulance came. Two pairs of quiet efficient hands prepared me for the journey to hospital, making me conscious for the first time of my right arm hanging at uncontrolled angles, and of my bloody, wet face. I thought of these kindly men as other people's fathers, on loan to those who were unable to look after themselves.

A golden light surrounded me, penetrating my eyelids which were torn and covered with blood and glass. This fact only registered in a fleeting way when the casualty nurse tried to wash my face, for thankfully, I was still insensible everywhere but in my thoughts, and even they were difficult to bring together.

"Where shall I cut your jumper?" the nurse asked.

"I don't mind," I said. Who cares, I thought.

"Who should we contact first? The surgeon or the ophthalmologist?"

The young doctor and nurse discussed their possible actions on my behalf. They worked in an atmosphere of unhurried normality. The questionnaire was filled in.

"How many cigarettes do you smoke a day? Did you have chickenpox as a child? Are you allergic to any drugs?"

The great energy it took to answer the questions responsibly suddenly dissipated, and as the nurse wrapped up my whole head, scrunchy glass, torn tissues and blood, I retreated beyond the light into my cocoon. I seemed to be only alive in my mind, and yet during that night as I slipped in and out of consciousness, I became more aware of driving, unrelenting pain.

New, tender voices accompanied me through that night, reassuring and always with me.

"You're going to be operated on at nine in the morning." This sentence became a beacon of release from this prison of pain. Soon, soon, I prayed, and then at last . . . I was in a void . . . a vacuum of real anaesthesia.

"Don't move your head if you can help. Try not to be sick if you possibly can. Breathe deeply and slowly — good girl."

Bottles and tubes are adjusted — my whole head is enclosed in bandages — only my mouth is free, which becomes dry with my breathing. Drifts of discomfort envelop me; injections send me floating; many footsteps come and go, the hands that accompany them tend my every need. My broken arm has plaster to my shoulder. I drink through a bent straw; bags support my head. My mother arrives from interstate, trying not to cry. A friend with her doesn't know what to say. My back is warm and safe on my sheepskin. I do not know what is wrong and I do not care. My body is now conscious, but my mind is not. I need to rest, and rest, and rest.

Slowly as the days pass, I wake to my public ward. Old ladies sing in their senility, calling for pans as babies cry for love — one dies in the bed next to me, and as activity increases as she moves towards her point of departure, I escape into sleep. I am near the staff desk, still watched over. That desk is the focus of my interest which fans out each day as patients wake in their beds, their voices calling to each other like birds in their separate trees, adjusting their wings to the winds of authority for the good of their health.

What freedom I felt when the drip was removed

and my nose unplugged. Only the bandages on my eyes remained. I could move a little and breathe comfortably. Sleep came easier so that day and night separated. The staff materialized, becoming individuals performing incessant tasks. And as I shed the trappings of the very ill, I too emerged from anonymity. The chief surgeon and I began a game. He would arrive, asking me in his lovely, warm voice if I knew who he was. I always recognized his voice, but could never remember his name. Flirting only with our voices, he made me feel a person . . . worth cherishing, as well as worth saving.

One evening a young doctor came to my bedside, gently brushing my hand and saying, "Hullo Maxene. Mind if I sit and talk to you for a few minutes? I'm Dr Meadows, Resident here."

"As you probably realize," Yes, I said to myself, he's here to discuss my future. "You went through the windscreen of your car. Do you remember exactly what happened?"

We swapped notes, and then he told me. The two compound fractures in my right arm would mend, but I could possibly lose my left eye and be blind in my right. It was too early to tell yet. "We must be optimistic but nevertheless be prepared for the worst." The scarring on my face would be extensive, but would heal. He told me how his wife had adjusted to her facial scarring, sustained in an accident during their honeymoon.

How could the hospital subject this junior medic to the ordeal of telling me such things? I wanted to comfort him like I had done with my mother, assuring him that I would be all right. Whatever happened, I would be all right.

After he had gone, everything seemed subdued and slow, as if waiting for me to feel the truth. I tried on a picture in my mind's eye of me being blind. There I was with all the paraphernalia of the handicapped — long cane, guide dog, dark glasses and an eye patch. I walked along being courageous, beautifully dressed, and oblivious of the passers-by pausing to pay homage with their glances, to one who was so young and so brave. Somehow it didn't ring true. I knew I would be all right. I would see, I felt sure. How, I asked myself, could an art teacher go blind? It didn't make sense.

The next day I battled with trying to use a pan while lying still on my back in bed. Sister Oakley, the charge sister, insisted that I could if I really tried. Nurses whistled, ran taps all over the ward, chattered nonchalantly by my side — all to no avail. Sister Oakley managed to be scathing in her silence. To my dismay she arrived that afternoon to remove the two hundred and twenty stitches from my face. She was so skilful and light in her touch, I fell asleep. If only she could direct that energy to support my efforts to bring my shocked nervous system into line, instead of bullying me.

During peak administration time a few days later, what seemed like a herd of hospital élite walked ceremoniously into the ward to circle casually around my bed. Most chatted in the background as Dr Clark, the ophthalmologist, stripped me of my final bandaging, saying, "Let's see how these eyes are going."

My face felt so vulnerable and so exposed. He bathed, snipped, and gently eased my eyes free. I became aware of the cool air on my lids and a soft registration of light in my right eyelid.

"Now," he said, matter-of-factly, "can you open your eyes?" My left eye was very sore behind a fresh patch. My exposed lid fluttered open with great effort. With assumed calm, I realized that I could not only see light, but light with a definite shape. My eyes streamed.

"Can you see anything?"

And in the silence I pointed to squares of yellow brightness and described them.

"Good," Dr Clark said. "They are clerestory windows. Can you see how many people are here?"

"It sounded as though an army was arriving," I replied. They laughed, breaking the unacknowledged tension for a second.

"I can only see vague shapes. It's as though I'm looking through a watery fish shop window with the lights out inside. I think there are eight or nine of you . . ."

I tried harder, bringing forth another stream of water from my eyes which Dr Clark gently wiped away.

". . . I'm pretty sure there are nine."

"There are nine of us," he said with contained pleasure. "Very good indeed. We'll leave this pad on for a few days yet, to let your eye become accustomed to light. These things can't be hurried." Their sedate footsteps drifted away into silence.

"That's great news," said Caroline, my favourite nurse, offering to read me a story.

"Yes . . . thank you," I said. Inside me, my breath seemed full and penetrating. I settled deep under covers, nursing my news behind my eye pads, secure in my recovered vision that was too precious to experience again that day. It had all been so controlled. There should have been pipes and drums and great ceremony, but here crises passed enmeshed in a simple routine; so commonplace they ceased to be remarkable.

Nevertheless, the most simple accomplishment gave me enormous pleasure. As soon as autocratic Sister Oakley took a few days' leave, I managed to unspasm my plumbing. My hair was washed for the first time, and just in time for my birthday I was allowed to sit up. What pampering and powdering I received that day! My colleagues sent me a deep sea green dressing gown — a froth of flowing colour that I could see. All day my pulse was awry. Now that the crisis was over, friends could come every visiting hour, eager to celebrate my optimism. It seemed that everyone I knew felt the relief from my shadows. They swarmed like spring bees by my bed that September, holding fragrant posies that most of them had picked themselves from their gardens, as though aware I had escaped not ever seeing them again.

The day came when I could get out of bed, not walking yet, mind you, but go for a wheelchair ride around the ward. Out came my birthday negligee, I put on my slippers, then a brief unstable stand by the bedside, and off we went on our visiting tour.

"Who would you like to visit first?" my driver asked.

"Mrs Bennett," I suggested. "She has had no visitors during my stay." From my own bed I had felt her loneliness and her shame each time her pan had arrived too late.

"Hullo, Mrs Bennett," I said, as we manoeuvred close so that I could see her from my new dark glasses. "I've been looking forward to meeting you."

"We are so pleased with your progress, my dear," she said.

Suddenly I realized that she was really studying my face. Its tinctured tracery of tiny new stitch marks and discoloured tracks of injury must have been quite a sight I suppose.

"Heavens!" she said, in tones she must have used for her Sunday School classes. "Will your face ever get better?"

"Yes," I said, as though she were speaking of someone else.

"That's good," she said, huffing back with relief into her pillow. "Because you'd never get a man to marry you with a face like that."

My chariot was wheeled around in great agitation and haste.

"Goodbye," I said over my swiftly retreating shoulder. "I'll see you later."

"It's OK," I told the sister quietly. "She's only voicing her concern. She just doesn't understand."

I realized without seeing myself, that the war might be over, but the pain still remained.

For the rest of my stay, the endless shifts of activity were punctuated with other people's highs and lows. My time was like that of a clock whose wind-up period is almost over, its ticking becoming so faint and fading that you hardly remember its going.

By contrast, the day I left hospital is sharp and stabbing in my memory. I was gorged with emotion — a cocktail of sad farewells and frightening expectation. Hugs and handshakes, and a trickle of goodbyes accompanied me from bedside to car. I was out of hospital. We edged our way into the noisy lines of Saturday morning traffic. Almost a season had passed since my last car ride. The stormy gusts of that misadventure were nowhere near me now.

The sun was gloriously hot. It prickled the skin on my arm through the open window, and the metal by my elbow sent a searing stream of light into my new sight. My closed eyes and sunglasses could not keep out the glare, but occasionally I peered through a tiny slit to catch small clues to my whereabouts. We turned a corner to enter the beach road.

"Thank goodness we're out of that traffic," said Jess. "You weren't nervous, I hope?" she added, letting out a deep breath and her clutch as I reassured her.

Strips of flickering shadows passed over us, and the moist smell of sea jostled in my nostrils with the hot tang of gum leaves overhanging the road. The wind came to meet my breath, filling my lungs like bellows — fanning every nerve of my body into raw, exquisite sensing.

"We're almost home." Jess said. Behind me in the hospital, my elderly friends would never know the touch of sun or moving air upon their faces; captives in their beds for all the days before they died. I might have been killed, I thought. Gone forever. Suddenly death lay between me and the sun. With a flash of insight I realized that, like an errant finger on a chopping block, life can be cut from you in an instant. I would always remember that. But now I was alive, miraculously alive.

Around the corner we drove, up the hill and under

the shelter of the carport, honking the horn loudly.

"At last," sighed Jess.

Almost immediately her mother handed me out of the car, through the doorway and into the cool dimness of the loungeroom. I could hardly see a thing in front of me and the soft light was protection for my adjusting vision.

"I'm glad you're here," Jess's mother said. Sheets of tears precipitated within me.

"I'm glad I'm here too," I said.

The room was full of the warmth of human activity, but it could not shield me from new knowledge. For twenty-six years, like a child I had accepted the inevitable rise of the sun each day. Now, like an Eve who has just eaten, I knew that I could not expect to be here every tomorrow to see it happen.

"Are you all right?" Jess asked. "Would you like to lie down for a while?"

"No," I said, collapsing onto a couch amongst the clutter of her mother's crochet. "I'll just sit down and catch my breath."

11. The waning of my public eye

Exactly a week before my car accident, almost to the hour, I sat discussing hopes and fears with two friends. Jess suggested that she was afraid of losing someone that she cared about and I told them of my fears. I felt that I was going to be asked to sacrifice, to give up for some reason, something that was very precious to me; like a young person still in the height of physical strength and not yet aware of any sense of mortality, I thought perhaps I might lose the use of my legs. Not to be able to run and to dance and to move freely and expressively, I thought, would be a terrible deprivation. Then on the following Saturday evening at about midnight, I had the car accident only two hundred yards from my destination, Jess's flat.

I confounded the medicos with my very swift recovery. I wanted to get back into the world as soon as possible. The sight in my right eye continued to improve, and in the left, eventually a tiny glimmer came in one corner, not really any use, but still a kind of window or aperture to the visual world. Vision gives you a secure feeling of being actually in the world. It is an easy kind of reality, one doesn't have to work for it. I even got to drive my car again. The first time I sat in it, this time fitted with seat belts, I had a strange feeling. It didn't look the same; everything was now second hand. There were chips out of the steering wheel and I was to discover, under the rubber mats, blood stains and spots where acid from the battery had spilt, but I was driving again and I drove for four years.

During that time I reached the peak of my teaching ability with the Education Department. I continued to be taken up very actively in the intellectual pursuits of the college. I drank in the conversations over lunch — discussions that students and academics have probably had for years. In my public working life, there was a great deal of satisfaction, but in my private, emotional life there was a sense of dryness, of being unsure and not finding my place. My relationships came and went, many of them turning into friendships. One relationship that lasted for quite some time, I think back on with a great deal of pain, for it should never have been any more than a supportive friendship. At the time it began I was still in hospital, and I was vulnerable. What I needed was an affectionate uncle or father, but instead this person, out of his own need, shifted the focus of our relationship to much more. I regret that still, and wish that I'd been mature and strong enough to rebuff the help that came with the unwelcome offer of adult love.

One afternoon coming home from college, as Jess and I were driving past the Geelong wool stores, I voiced a sudden feeling that came over me. It felt like an emotional fog descending.

"Jess," I said, "I've got that feeling again."

"What feeling?"

"That feeling that something horrible is going to happen."

It was not long after this, I drove to Warrnambool one evening to pick Jess up after her grandfather's funeral. It was a very long drive; when I sat eating dinner with the family, I felt very tired but thought no more of it. On the way back, the heater failed in the car and the road was covered with wreaths of fog — real fog this time. I drove as swiftly as I could with my wheels flanking the white lines on the road. I felt that visibility was very poor indeed. When I reached the flat, I felt cold to my marrow so to help me to get warm, I got into a very hot bath. It was only later that I realized that I was in fact, suffering from a physical shock. When I climbed into bed and put on my reading light, the print in the book was speckled with small black dots. It seemed to be shifting and very small indeed. My eyes watered with the effort of reading it. That evening, beside my bed, I had four books. It was the last time I would ever read normal print and it seemed unfair that I should not have been able to savour it, a little as a condemned person savours their last breakfast. Which book would I have chosen? The small introduction to the Greek philosophers, Virginia Woolf's short stories with "The Death of a Moth", Pasternak's *Doctor Zhivago*, or the book on Australian architecture? The deprivation of independent reading was to last for quite a number of years. So many years, I find it hard to believe.

Great changes came about the following day. I drove my car to the ophthalmologist's surgery later that day in what seemed to be bright moonlight. When he tested my vision, he discovered that within twenty-four hours, I had lost an enormous amount and that my visual field was suddenly severely restricted. I would have to go to Melbourne for tests and also to have an operation for a detached retina. A small amount of glass, not detectable at the time of the accident, had worked in behind the retina and had gradually torn it. For some time that tiny tear must have held, but then, with the changing pressures of normal physiological ebbs and flows within the eye, the strain had been too much and the retina had suddenly given way. The thought that I would miss work for something like three months was a most terrible shock to me. I went outside to sit in my car. I saw everything about me with an abnormal clarity — the red gravel drive seemed to stand out in enormous contrast to the white trunk of a beautiful gum. Every bush, every flower seemed to imprint its shape and colour in my eye. I've rarely seen quite as consciously as in those moments. It was as though I already knew that my vision was not to last and that these precious lookings at a most beautiful earth were to be brief. To be savoured.

A few days later I spent the whole morning being tested in the Eye Hospital. At about midday, Professor Crock and one of his most senior students sat with me to consider the various aspects of my case. I had been by now prepared for an operation and a long convalescence, but I was little prepared for the news that my retina had quite a large cyst in it. To operate would be quite dangerous. My eye would most probably haemorrhage and so obliterate the little sight that I had. There was a possibility of trying to operate and Professor Crock suggested that I discuss it with my family. Very firmly, I told him that the responsibility for such a decision could not be handed over to anyone else, that if I consequently lost my vision completely, I would not allow others to share in the feeling of being responsible. It was a decision that I must make for myself. He seemed to talk to me a little differently after that and this was the first of many wonderful meetings with the Professor; he didn't just treat my eyes, but spoke to me as a total being — considering that what was happening to me as a result of my visual difficulties, was just as important as the physical condition of my eye.

I was taken back to a ward but unfortunately, my history was left behind so that no one knew the news that I had just been told. How long it would be before I was totally blind was absolutely unpredictable, but that was certainly what would eventuate. I sat up in bed with nurses scurrying about with my late lunch and finally when some unsuspecting nurse asked me if I would like cream or custard on my sweets — that decision seemed so irrelevant to my situation — I just burst into tears.

"What's wrong?" asked the nurse. I managed to tell her I'd had some bad news and suggested that she ask the doctor. I could not stop crying.

"Don't upset yourself" said a senior sister who came to intervene. "Don't upset yourself. Stop crying, otherwise you'll make yourself sick."

If only they'd let me fill the pillow with tears of grief and disappointment and feelings of strange fulfilment. Was it a fulfilment of a prophecy, of a superstition, or a sense of things following a rightful course? "Please can I have a bath?" I asked as they tried to give me a sedative, "I just need a bath and a sleep."

At least the bath was private. I lay there in the water feeling like a child, escaping from a harsh world where people told you you must be so brave and not whimper when you were hurt in the depths of yourself. Once in the bath, I could no longer cry. I thought back to the time in hospital when Neil had come to see me and made it perfectly plain, in his business-like fashion, that I no longer had a place in his life. My logical mind told me that of course, that had already happened. I'd known when I'd gone to Geelong that we would eventually part. I knew also that it was a mis-match, but I was to be reminded in hospital that not only was I unworthy, as someone from a working class background, to become a member of his family, but as a handicapped person, an unthinkable one. Well, here I was, going blind. How many others would reject me because of it? How could I battle with the sense of still being me? How could I let people know that I hadn't changed? The next months and years were to see great difficulties and some small triumphs. I spent a lot of time proving my strength, showing that I could still be an efficient and independent person.

That evening, Professor Crock called in to see me and suggested that for the time being, they should not do any investigations and risk impairing the partial vision I had at that time. He also suggested that I go home to Geelong and have my ophthalmologist there operate on the post-operative cataract that was covering my left eye. There was only a fifty-fifty chance of that working but it was worth the try.

That operation was a missed chance, a textbook situation of haemorrhage. I had the operation late one afternoon and early the next morning, at about five, the night sister came to give me my sponge in bed. I was still very sleepy from the anaesthetic and as she lifted my head, I half awoke, saying, "Please don't touch my head. I've had a cataract removed." She insisted that no such thing had happened and that I'd only had a needle. As I persisted she went to look in the book. When she returned, she said, "Well, it's not in the book, dear, so you must have only had a preliminary." As she moved me this way and that, I felt out of control. By the end of the washing, she realized that the anaesthetic was still showing its hand and that perhaps after all I may have had an operation. This sister was in fact, a very skilful and very sincere person and I suppose to her the thought that some mistake could be made in the records was unthinkable, but the mistake had been made. My head, that morning, should have been left quiet and undisturbed and so, quite predictably, on the third day after the operation, my eye haemorrhaged very badly. My doctor was not contactable and all during that day, the pain in my eye increased. Visitors came during the afternoon and I found it almost impossible to concentrate on them. That evening I asked that someone else see me, but again this didn't seem to be possible. It was only a small private hospital and so doctors tended to have their weekends like everyone else. Sunday evening, I was in a world of my own, steeped in the pain. My doctor arrived and in a great flurry of distress and tension, I had injections in an effort to save the eye itself. Of course with this event, there was no thought of my ever having sight in that eye. A fifty-fifty chance had fallen on the wrong side. For ten weeks I lay in that hospital draining the haemorrhage, treating my bed almost as a cocoon of comfort and retreat.

The accident had been a sudden and shocking event but as soon as I began to get well and my future looked optimistic, friends flocked about me. This time, the situation was quieter and had a sense of foreboding. It seemed that most people tried to ignore what I was going through. Only the more solid families, whose sense of duty perhaps overcame their feelings, came to see me. Jess and I had shared a flat for several years by this time. Now I hardly saw her. It is difficult to handle one's own pain but even more difficult to forgive and understand when another is unable to overcome their own feeling, to give you at least a small amount of support. Her action of running away from what she saw as a most terrible future, has been a rare response to what has happened to me. Most times, I have been able to assist those whose shock is at first great and their courage faltering, but with Jess we were separated by work and hospital, so that choice was never given me.

In contrast there was Father's reaction to my inevitable blindness. He did not know it was scientifically impossible but he offered me one of his eyes as a transplant. This supreme act of generosity left me speechless and deeply moved. It compensated a great deal for the rejection I had felt.

In the last months of my life in Geelong, I lived in a kind of reduced way, becoming increasingly aware of the new skills it would be necessary to learn to make my life full again. On one occasion, a blind man with a guide dog came to speak to the college assembly. When he was led into the hall with the truly sightless eyes that some blind people have, my heart sank and it took all my courage to keep my equanimity in front of the crowd. As he spoke, I realized I did not like him; the thoughts and ideas which he presented were not going to be mine. There was a sense of bitterness which was unspoken, but nevertheless present in his manner of speaking, but it was not the dislike which disturbed me. It was that knowledge of lack of independence. Even with the dog, there was a sense of a lost child about him and I vowed that there would never be that atmosphere about me, no matter what happened.

In January, when I knew that I could no longer continue with my job, even though at this stage they had been enormously generous to me, I was offered a job in Melbourne, helping to prepare a new version of the art and craft course — the section on fabric and threads. I'd already done experimental work in that direction, and to help to formulate this section of the course was a challenge. Living in Melbourne would also enable me to learn the skills that I was bursting to get on with. I had already been in touch with the braille library and was learning braille on the job, on a six-week course. Contact with the young, totally blind teacher, who had been a sighted art teacher, helped me in my attitude to blind people. By March the following year, I was in a flat and beginning a whole new life. Travelling on public transport was something I'd never enjoyed. Not to be able to get into my car and zip here and there at a whim, was at first an unexpressed but very real frustration. I could only just see numbers on the trams, and one evening in winter, I shopped too late in the city, and when I got out of the tram, it was pitch dark. My particular kind of partial vision made me virtually totally blind, once the sun was set.

There was no-one about and in the rush of first foolhardy courage, by judging the lights of the cars, which were the only things I could see, I managed to cross the busy road. Once on the other side, I could not find the footpath. Round the corner on my left, a car drove quite fast. I had gone into the street, and was walking down the side of the road. I walked across to the footpath and heard some footsteps in front of me. I followed them right down the path, bumping into the bushes or the fence as I went. When we came to the last street to cross in front of the flats, this woman paused and I asked her a question about the entrance to the flats. She responded very coolly but somehow I managed to follow her across the road and to find my flat door — at last there was some lighting. It was only when I got inside I realized she probably thought I was drunk because of my unusual method of walking, very tentatively, and not quite straight. I picked up the telephone and rang a friend in a flurry of contained emotion; for now that it was over, the feelings came. There were many such experiences in those early days — travelling was never a small or easy feat for me.

For quite a number of years, I managed to present myself as a sighted person. Even with a limited amount of vision in the day time, I could do things quite well. I could pick up a couple of visual clues and fill in my imaginative picture from previous experience. I'd always been extremely observant so now that skill was used in my efforts to see in my own mind.

This new picturing of the world about me enabled me to predict what was going on and effectively take part — with as little guesswork and gaucheness as possible. Sometimes I was slow, even difficult, for to make a mistake in front of others and not to care takes a particular lack of pride. I felt happy to do things differently inside me, within my perception, but I wanted to appear to others as a person who seemed to manage her physical world in the same way as everyone else did.

In August of that year, I bought a small house. This was a great joy to me. It was a little cottage, most attractive, with dark inside walls. I could turn on the electric lights and keep out of the sunlight, thus protecting the partial vision, which was diminished by the effects of the sun. I had taught myself to touch-type using a Pitman's book. I was efficient enough to write letters, but the typewriter and I have had an uneasy relationship. The absolute discipline of doing exactly what the type says just doesn't seem to fit with my experimental and creative nature. I also had several mobility lessons and my braille continued. Unfortunately, the first braille book I ever got from the library was one of Greek history. It was very old and almost rubbed out. The Greek names were so long and unfamiliar, that the book became a daunting project.

At that time the welfare agencies were the only dispensers of audio library materials. The talking book was considered an opiate for the aged. I was still not fluent enough in braille to enjoy reading a book in that medium and so for as long as I had any vision, however limited, I used it. For two years I waited for a talking book. For someone who had been an avid reader, this was some kind of purgatory. I knew that the waiting list was long and that my need was considered less urgent than those whose life was severely restricted by their age and illness. Nevertheless, it was as though a part of my life had been cut away from me and I felt it keenly. Every few months or so I would appear at the welfare officer's door asking if I was any closer to getting a book. He always jollied me along, expressing the idea that I lived such a full and active life that there was plenty else to do. There was, but it didn't make up for loss of reading. When I had to go into hospital for an unsuccessful investigation of the cyst in the right eye, a blind friend mentioned to me that hospital patients were never denied access to a talking book and machine. I applied, and got it. I sat up in hospital and 'read' Thomas Hardy's *Far from the Madding Crowd*. I can still smell the dusty, subtle, indefinable smell of that machine and its book, and as the words came into my wide open self, they felt like a bath of warm water on an open wound. I was supposed to return the machine and books as soon as I returned from hospital. I did not. I felt that my need was as great as anyone's and that two years was long enough to go without what seemed to me an essential part of my life. It would have taken a brigade of soldiers to have retrieved that machine from me. That experience, more than any other, determined me to be active in bringing about library services for print-handicapped people, based on what was available for those who could see. In the late seventies, I took part in the National Federation of Blind Citizens' efforts in this direction and, still later, served on the committee of the Braille and Talking Book Library, in the hope of seeing this principle implemented in the service delivery of the library itself.

For as long as I had a little vision, I continued to use it. I wrote recipes in large print with a felt pen. I bought white crockery to sit on my dark benches and this contrasting of colours was very useful for me. I could put a white page on a dark bench and then a dark object on top so that I could see it more clearly. There were many tricks that I picked up along the way — how to know clothes were turned the right way, how to keep shoes in pairs, and I trained myself to be more efficient and detailed in my organization. When I came in from work, the keys had to be put in a particular place. In my usual human frailty I sometimes lost them and then there was a terrible scurry. Looking or searching for a lost object was the most frustrating thing of this period. It was a little like cleaning; one could not simply pick out the dirty spots and clean them up. Every clean was a spring clean.

In September I took over a job I'd been offered at the RVIB (Royal Victorian Institute for the Blind), teaching art and craft to visually handicapped people. For some time I'd been dissatisfied with keeping on my own old life in its changed fashion. I felt I needed a whole new direction. So without the loss of one day's work I changed from an Education Department teacher with all the status that my work had achieved to that of a handicapped person working in an institution. My wages were halved. I found it very difficult in this situation to keep the knowledge of my own worth. The Institute was run on business lines rather than educational ones and this increased my difficulties. The work itself was extremely demanding, for every student had to be assessed and given work that was entirely suitable for him or her. This drain on my creativity became increasingly difficult to keep up with. I enjoyed the work enormously and made contact that was very personal with each client. By Friday night I was exhausted. Often I would walk in at my door at five o'clock, throw my clothes by the side of the bed and sleep until nine or ten. An apple and a drink would keep me going and I would sleep again until eight the following morning. Every ounce of my concentration was now being used in an effort to continue in a way that I had done when I could see. I still cooked, I ironed, I washed, and I lived on my own to prove that I was still independent. There were times during the next few years when friends came to stay, and one of the joys of this time was that a number of my past students arrived on my door step deciding to adopt me and to include me in their youthful frivolities. And so on the one hand there was this very difficult, in some ways rewarding, work to be done, new perceptions to be collated and a whole new me to be integrated. On the other hand, in my social life there was great entertainment. It was a great wonder to me that I made new friends, and although the first year was a very solitary, lonely one, from then on Carter's Avenue became a kind of shelter for the many young people who were not rushing into marriage or single relationships, but who were enjoying life in a kind of group situation. My cultural life really flowered — plays, films, concerts and parties. I didn't enjoy parties, only the ones I gave myself, and these were flamboyant, crazy affairs, of far too many people crammed into a small space with lots of noise and laughter.

After the highly academic and rather conventional flavour of my working life in Geelong, this happy-go-lucky sort of adventurous existence was refreshing. For the first time in my life I dressed exactly as I pleased. People would often not realize that I was only partially sighted and once they did they found the subject fascinating. Talking of such things allowed me to cut through the frivolity and the trivial nature of much social intercourse. There were many important and lasting relationships made at this stage. There was one person I was particularly fond of. Younger than I was, very vital, a little zany, good looking and utterly charming. It was more an infatuation than a lasting love, but I would not have missed that relationship for anything. It was a tempestuous and difficult affair. One of those brilliant and fascinating phases — not meant to last, but which I remember with tenderness and poignancy.

In my work at the Institute I had tried to assist those who had partial vision to use it more fully. People who had never painted before did it with great enjoyment and accepted their sight as having an integrity of perception of its own. As well, I wanted those who suddenly lost vision to be able to convert from using sight to using all of the other senses in an easy and efficient way. To help me with this I decided to do a six-month study tour overseas. This was a most marvellous trip, but by the time I got home I had very little vision left. I'd learnt very little, but it had given me rest and relaxation and filled my store of experience enormously.

Diminishing vision was for me, like veil after veil descending, obscuring the clarity of shape and making colours indistinguishable from each other. Yellows and pinks blended together, then blues, purples and greens, until finally I could see only red. The last visual pictures I had were an amorphous mixture of sepia tints and textures which my imagination had to interpret. With every change of visual perception there were fresh adjustments to make. I lived with the possibility of my remaining sight going overnight. To live with the expectation of waking the following morning to total blindness was like living on the edge of a precipice. Even so, when the veils became too dense to see through, there was a feeling of greater security and relief. When you are at last totally blind you are no longer faced with the unrealistic expectations of others and you yourself know where you are. I could then concentrate on developing my remaining senses. This tuning of sound, smell and touch added new perceptions which I found amazing. At first, sensing objects from a few feet away seemed to be some sort of magic which some very able blind people perform. I was delighted one evening when I stepped out of a car to realize, without the aid of usual sensing, that I was standing very close to the trunk of a tree and that its branches and leaves formed a canopy above my head. People too were discernible in this way, although some drew so close within themselves that I could hardly "feel" them. Others with stronger, more dynamic personalities were easy to find in my new field of inner seeing. I discovered too, that I could sit in an armchair and sense the sun filling the room, expanding it with warmth and vitality, and then "see" the walls retract again as the source of the brilliant light was obscured by cloud. The sensing of atmosphere is sometimes described by people as feeling vibrations, but that seems to me to be a narrow version of a most intriguing ability we can all cultivate if only we allow it to happen. In an everyday sense, we can experience it when we walk into a person's home for the first time: before there is activity or interaction to colour the immediate picture we have as soon as we walk through the door. An empty house can still bear the stamp of the family who has just vacated it. As time went on, this impressionistic inner viewing of the world about me became a rich source of satisfaction and wonder. All through the era of changing visual perception, one part of me watched the process with absolute fascination, as though monitoring the experience for future reference, although I knew this to be an illogical conclusion. This period of partial vision spanned the vital, physically expressed part of my life and the more difficult but profound inner life that was to come.

A contemplation: A look at blindness

"Does she take sugar?" they ask my friend as if I cannot hear.

"How does she manage?" they say as if I cannot move.

"Can you dress yourself?"

"Who buys your clothes?"

"Who will look after you in your old age?"

"Your husband must be a marvellous man."

"Surely you didn't make that crochet jacket? Someone must have helped you."

An observer sees the picture and traces its outlines and details with the eyes. To be blind means experiencing — touching, sensing, feeling, being, doing. To see and not to see are the two sides of perception, for not to see does not mean not to perceive. It simply means a different way of looking. To be blind is to be born again into the same world, but with a different angle of your camera.

*In fact, to be precise, you have no camera at all —
you have to live your life. This great adventure, this
penetration of existence to a layer not previously experienced, is exciting and sometimes scarey. Of course there
is the grief of things once seen — the language of eyes;
the gestures of hand and leg and smile; pictures; the
colour of flowers as they are in the flowers and not just
as they live in my present imagination; the sight of an
open landscape with its nuances which come from the
relationship of movements of earth, sun, moon and stars.
But soon I was to learn that all of these things were the
tonal qualities of what I could experience in essence if
I were prepared to open myself like a flower to the sun.
If I try to look at the sun with my old eyes I will be
truly blind and if I do not drink in what is about me,
I will perish.*

12. Ben and Katie

In late August 1971, I went skiing with a group of
blind people. I was in the process of licking my
wounds after the end of my previous relationship
but found with great surprise that I was viewing
another male with great interest. On the trip to the
ski resort Ben, a partially sighted man a little older
than myself, was most attentive. He knew exactly
what to do. How to show me my chair, how to
indicate eating utensils and various other small
things which I normally had to fumble about for
myself. I'd met him before, but now I really saw

him for the first time. We laughed and giggled together over spilling our peas and doing silly things
with the bread that sat on the side of the counter
lunch. I told him stories of how I'd tried to eat a
quarter of a lemon and a huge garnish of parsley the
first time I'd ever gone out to dinner with a man
after beginning to lose sight. He understood the
laughter that hid the embarrassment and the feelings
of shame.

He'd known blind people since he was a child.
He'd been sent to the RVIB school after it was found
not possible for him to see the board at an ordinary
school. He had many heart-rending stories to tell
me of those early days. During the war the school
had moved to Olinda and there they'd roamed the
hills, got dirty and explored like every other child.
It was the saving of their normality. The totally
blind children always felt that the children with
some vision were really their servants. Very few
partially sighted people actually got to university.
All the accent was on the totally blind and on braille.
He knew braille well.

There was much to discuss and enjoy in his
company. At the end of the trip we'd made arrangements to see his race-horse run in the country. We
had wished to spend more time together but every
time he assisted me from one place to another one
of the official mobility officers interrupted us. We
laughed about that later. Several weeks later a car
load of us went to see his horse run and it won. We
hugged each other and jumped up and down with
joy. All the way there and all the way back during
that long country run, Ben and I talked. We stopped
at a country pub. One of the party introduced us to

the hotel keeper and it was suggested that we have a bottle of champagne. Amid all that group celebration Ben quietly indicated that a cup of tea would restore us in a way that was necessary. I felt the same but would have given in to the champagne — I then decided that he was just the person to spend the rest of my life with.

From our next meeting till the day we were married we were inseparable. It was like coming home. This tall, gentle, but very certain person gave me a sense of being wanted and needed and loved in a way never before given. I discovered that he was enormously strong in his resolve, despite his usually easy-going demeanour.

Within three months of our first going out together we were married. We escaped to Sydney, away from the tangled situations of our families, and there in a quiet ceremony Ben and I pledged ourselves to each other. The few friends who were there threw frangipani over us and the day was filled with bright summer light. All the relationships that had gone before now seemed irrelevant. Ben and I were mates in the very real sense of the word. Although at this time we thought we couldn't love each other more it was not true. The years ahead drew us together with a deepening and more tender love for each other than I had ever thought possible. Even now as I write Ben's name I have a feeling of warmth flow through me and a deep sense of gratitude for his being.

We set off the day after we were married to see my grandmother in Mudgee. I wanted to bring together the two people who were the sentinels of my early life and of a future whose prospect now filled me with great happiness. I had a deep unexpressed longing to bring the riches that had been a part of my very young life into the life that Ben and I were to share together. It seemed a kind of growing up. I would no longer wait for life to bring things to me, but now had the responsibility with Ben of actually building the colour, the texture and the meaning of our existence together.

In the first month of my pregnancy I was very much afraid I would lose the child that grew within me. I had longed for this experience of womanhood and to have the privilege of helping a child grow to adulthood. By the fourth month my mind was at peace and so I began to enjoy myself. Like cats when they are expecting, I lay in the spring sun and slept the afternoon through. Life was as simple as it could be and then suddenly I became very active. This time I was like the birds. I began to nest.

Ben and I shifted from Carter's Avenue to a house more suitable for a child. It had a large, safe backyard and throughout the house there was a free movement of air and lots of sunlight pouring in. The windows in the bedrooms let in the morning sunshine and in the afternoons there was the bright light of sunset through a sunroom. Just outside these windows a twenty-foot cumquat tree blossomed and fruited all the year round. The garden was exactly right for a child. There were nooks and crannies and sixteen fruit-bearing trees, including a fig tree — later on a swing hung from its branches and beneath its friendly foliage a sand pit invited all kinds of truly imaginative play. During the early summer months there was much to be done. I cleaned, rearranged and adorned the house for the baby's coming. I would stand by the cradle with its blankets in a dust proof package, wondering what the child would be like who was soon to lie there. It didn't seem to matter if it was a boy or a girl, although I tended to think that it was going to be a boy. To try and imagine the personality of a little being before it is born is an amazing exercise. Ben and I went through the usual pre-natal preparations. We watched a film about a birth just a few weeks before our own. We sat together holding hands deeply moved by what is such a common event, but steeped with enormous meaning and effect on the people who take part in it.

When our baby was slightly overdue, because of my age, Dr Gallant threatened to induce the birth the following morning. On the way home in the taxi I had several small contractions. In the hospital that night they were erratic, but still there; at about ten I was woken by a very large pop as my water broke. And thus began a most exciting time in our lives. At 4.30 the following morning, much to the surprise of the sister, I delivered a baby girl.

She came into the world with a great rush. Two contractions, fast upon each other, brought her little head into the open air and soon after her little body followed. I immediately put my hands on her as she was laid on my stomach. Don't touch her the sister said, you're not sterile. What nonsense they talk. I touched her anyway. Shortly after, she was wrapped in a rug and in my arms, crying intermittently and sneezing as she had swallowed a little amniotic fluid. I soothed her, talking to her all the while, touching her with absolute wonder.

Hospital was hard work. I asked that I might have

a lot of contact with little Kate so that I could bond with her very early, for perhaps the two of us might have difficulties which we had yet not foreseen. I fed her in the middle of the night, changed her nappy and bathed her each day. For some reason that was never made clear to me the sister in charge of the nursery suggested to Dr Gallant that I wean Kate. I was appalled. It was against everything that I thought should happen. They explained that a previous blind patient had bottle-fed her baby, her husband preparing the formula for her each night and leaving the bottles in the refrigerator to be used when needed. I asked with great sincerity that they help me to continue feeding Kate for it was something that I would not give up. In the next few days I discovered that she had been bottle-fed before she came to me and was also test-weighed when every other baby born on the same day was well past that. These were but few of the subtle ways in which the staff continually indicated their disbelief in my ability to look after my child. I had examined this question for myself and decided that, since I had proved I could look after myself, with intelligent preparation I was perfectly capable of taking care of my child. Every evening when Ben arrived I was, if not tearful, on the verge of it. In the midst of the bank of flowers and the stream of well-wishers who came I was miserable. I was being treated just as someone handicapped. They weren't truly seeing me. I knew that as soon as I got home I would be all right and I was.

Kate was the most perfect little baby. Her skin had a pink blush and she had quite a deal of hair. She was tiny like a small flower, her fingers and feet moving toward the air. As Ben and I walked through our front door with Katie we were overflowing with a sense of not just love, but of immense responsibility. We had a sacred task ahead of us, the bringing up of a tiny human being. The first thing I did was to feed her so that she felt secure and then she slept for four hours straight. Ben changed her nappy that evening for the first, but not the last time, and with this first act he was as involved with her as ever I was. This sharing of Kate's daily life deepened the tenderness between Ben and me, giving our marriage a different aspect as a result of our now being three.

As Kate began slowly to wake from the dreamy state of babyhood, it was quite evident that she was an individual in her own right and this we both respected. I often sat in the sunroom after I had fed her, with her asleep on my knees, watching the slight breeze through the window touching her thistledown hair and I wondered what life would bring to her. These thoughts were bitter sweet and I cannot imagine any parent loving or appreciating a child as much as I did then. Every single day was a first time not just for Kate, but for me also. As she began to grow I saw the world with absolutely fresh eyes. The wonder of seeing something, doing something, achieving something, thinking something, for the very first time in the whole of your life is just so obvious that its significance is often overlooked. As soon as she was able to crawl, off she would go in the garden, picking up flowers, smelling them with delight, laughing out loud as she touched their soft petals. Pieces of bark, stones and leaves were picked up and examined with absolute scrutiny and then put aside as if they no longer existed.

I can remember buying her her first sandals. When we got home she got them out of the box and began to play with them. Both Ben and I were about to take them from her to put them away safely but then realized that her play was in deep earnest. It was, in fact, learning work. She managed to put them on — on the wrong feet, but at least on — and made a good job of getting the straps into the buckles. It was a good lesson for us and from then on we always examined our position before we said no.

Kate somehow knew from the beginning that I could not see and simply took it in her stride. The first time I gave her something solid to eat, she helped to guide the spoon with her two minute fingers, holding the handle just above the bowl, next to mine. Breast feeding Kate had been for me a spiritual sharing of my body and my self which had satisfied my wish to give to my child as much as I was capable of. When she suddenly decided to wean herself, I got the taste of the highly independent and strong little girl that she was to become.

She talked before she walked, I suppose realizing that her world could best be managed in a verbal fashion in our household. She delighted us with her clear, bright little voice and her efforts, when she was not quite two, to speak huge words with great deliberation and enjoyment, words such as "incidentally" or "eventually". Her voice had a singing quality, which seemed to me to express her delight with the world, and so far as I can remember she could sing from the first time she tried. Maybe we could have been accused of being doting parents, besotted with our roles of parenthood. Nevertheless we understood that children come to us as gifts. "They are not of us, but they come through us," as it says in *The Prophet*. We were able to leave Kate quite free to develop herself in her own way. We were guardians of an emerging and unique human being. I look back at the first two years we had together and my feeling is that it was some kind of idyll. Ben and I, through our precious child, had shared a child's garden with the same sense of wonderment that we must have had at her age. An intense, deep thankfulness lies within me for the fact of Kate coming to us. Within me a well of tenderness filled and overflowed. It was almost exquisite in its intensity, and much richer in essence than the feelings of compassion and empathy I had previously experienced.

13. A lump in my breast

A lump in my breast. "I found a lump in my breast Elizabeth, and I hardly dare go to the doctor."

"I think this lump should be looked at by a specialist," says the doctor.

"This lump doesn't seem to be serious at this stage," says the specialist. "Just keep an eye on it."

During the next two months the lump becomes hard like a walnut and is very painful. At night I cup a hand on the left side of my breast so that I can sleep on my side. Eventually I have to face going back to the specialist.

"This lump will have to be investigated," says the specialist.

Ben is shocked. I have a sense of timelessness. A sense of my lifetime being a term, a short space. Am I being dramatic? Can I afford to think of my life as following the natural course of my dying of old age, or must I now think of this as being the beginning of the last stage of my life?

Ben and I drive from the surgery, two separate people, locked into our own fears, too full of pain to speak of it or to reach out to each other. Kate is oblivious.

I buy special nighties for the hospital with very large, easy openings. Kate plays with them so that I won't look strange to her in hospital.

Someone says, "If the lump is painful it's probably all right."

Someone else says, "Don't worry, most lumps are not carcinogenic."

I feel as though a dark cloak is hovering about me ready to fall on to my shoulders. Everything I do is difficult. It's as if I have to pull myself out of the mire to be able to do the everyday things. Kate is like a fragile, beautiful piece of my life that I hardly dare leave sight of. And at night I drink in the fragrance of Ben's warmth and love him as though they are the last minutes.

How will I know when I wake up if I've had the mastectomy or not? Will the bandages tell me? The anaesthetist replies, "The bandages will hardly be different. But don't worry, dear, I'll tell you before I leave."

A night of strange uneasy sleep, cap and gown in the morning, fuzzy injection-induced floating, touching my breast for the last time? Then oblivion. Where is my consciousness? Where do I go? Do they lift my breast and cut it cleanly off with a sword?

Someone shakes my shoulder vigorously. "Wake up. Wake up Mrs Hewitt. We've had to take your breast."

"Thank you," I say, not forgetting my manners.

A long and drugged sleep. Ben and Graeme sit by my side. Stricken and trying not to show it. Reaching me with their love. I drift in and out of the room.

Where is my breast now? Burning in some incinerator or laid out coldly in some laboratory? Have I lost my breast to save my life? I have a sense of being pruned, but for what? Several days pass. Drainage tubes come out, bandages are removed and there is my scar: a thin clean line runs down my chest and around in an arc up towards my underarm. My chest looks like that of a young boy. I show the scar to friends who come. I want them to feel better about me. Joan comes home from Queensland knowing that someone is ill. She cries in the car when Stan tells her. She knows as I know that there is much ahead.

Friends cried round my bed. I talked excitedly in a way that makes me feel very much alive. When they are gone I am rent with perspiration and very tired.

Kate comes almost every day to see me and sits on the bed, a little round ball of warm winter clothing, and I love her dearly and long to be home.

Within a fortnight Ben picks me up, and when I

go home he and Kate put a record on, and Kate tells me it's to make me feel better. She wants to sit on my knee, but her little elbows digging into my chest to find a right position hurt me and I find it necessary to place her beside me on the couch. She is too young to sit beside me, she should still be cradled in my arms.

I have no energy. I cry easily. I can't get out of a chair. Everything is such a job. And yet I struggle on. I cook better than I've ever cooked in my life. Wanting to nourish and to share with everyone I love, something I've created. Then I meet Marlene, a homoeopath. Self-taught and a deeply spiritual person. I begin on Bach drops and from that day I have no more tachycardia.

Nevertheless Marlene suggests I see a friend of hers called Peter who could help me unlock some of the secret needs I have.

I talk to him on the phone. He has a fresh, clear, young voice. "You sound," he says "as though you are carrying a burden too heavy for one. Shall we try to shoulder it together?" I say yes and feel great relief.

Therapy begins.

During these months, Peter and I laid the foundation for what was to be a fascinating and crucial kind of work. We needed to build trust and a method of working which suited us both. There was much to get to know before the real work could begin. It was during that winter that I began to have pain in my chest, along the line of my scar. I mentioned it to the doctor but he didn't think it was anything more than a particular condition of the scar tissue. One afternoon, on my way to a neighbour, a searing, cutting pain sent me to my knees. It diminished slightly but did not go away.

I was sent in to the doctor again and this time he found a substantial lump folded in amongst the engorged scar tissue. It was difficult to come to terms with this blow. I'd had three years of being free of cancer and hope was bright for our future. We had built a house close to a school we had specially chosen for Kate. It was a house which was to express all of my taste, all of my needs, and all that I wanted to share with my family and friends. It was to be a new beginning. Nine days before we were to shift I was in hospital having the lump removed. The only bright spot was my overhearing of a conversation between the matron and my surgeon.

"You are worse than Dame Nellie Melba", she said to him, "How many more times are you going to come back?"

"Oh, I'm off tomorrow," he said. He was going to holiday in Honolulu. "But I just could not pass over this woman to anyone else. I have known her for some time and I felt I must operate on her myself."

The care that was in that voice warmed me considerably. Actually, I never saw him again as he died suddenly during the following year and I was passed over to other doctors who were more versed in oncology.

The weekend I came home to recover was black indeed. I had news that a close friend who had come to help me when Kate first came home from hospital, had died from cancer on the Friday evening. She had died about the same time as I had had my lump removed. Peg had loved Kate and she and I had grown to cherish each other as very dear friends. She had come as a council help, but instead of the regulation three hours of assistance, we spent the whole day together, working, listening to music, having a prolonged lunch and enjoying Kate.

In preparation for the shift, I sat in a chair, packing one-handed into a tea chest which Ben positioned for me each morning. He packed into the small hours of the night. I felt cheated of what should have been a really joyous looking forward to new beginnings.

The past was still affecting the future in a way that was not good.

In October I went to Peter McCallum for ray treatment every working day for four weeks. I took supplementary vitamins and minerals and I ate like a horse. Apart from the fact that it was very tiring and depleting, I managed it very well. I was never sick and my skin stood up to the burning quite well. I travelled the nineteen miles into the city in the Red Cross bus and once in there, Eileen met me in the waiting room to sit and talk while we went through the boring procedures that surrounded the actual treatment. I was very grateful for this sharing, because sitting there in solitude for long periods of time would have been quite destructive and I would have taken into myself some of the atmosphere which surrounded me. At that time I was very open and vulnerable. Eileen acted as a bulwark. She only missed two days in those four weeks.

I decided that I should meditate in an effort to make full use of the ray treatment. I wished to spiritualize it. As soon as the door clanged shut and I waited for the zinging sounds of the actual ray, I began to meditate. I built pictures of healing experiences, the cleansing that goes on in nature, the work of the wind and the rain and regeneration. On one occasion I didn't need to build such a picture — one came as bright and as clear and as physically visual as an actual experience could be. I saw a most perfect garden. The air was bright with light and pure, as pure as you could imagine air could be. Flowers were vivid in their colour and vivacious in their movement. The flowers were sometimes recognizable, but overall I had the experience of drinking in beauty that was perfect, absolutely unadulterated, and beyond the inevitability of decay. I was to walk in this garden on many occasions in the future. It became a source of inspiration and a place of spiritual clarity.

On another occasion when for some reason I was a little uneasy during my meditation, an enormous arm came out and over my body as a kind of protection. The next day, the staff showed me the shape of the actual ray machine. It was, in fact, a physical facsimile of what I had seen in my meditation.

As soon as the ray treatment was over, I began to strengthen again and I also began really to enjoy our house. Light flooded in from every direction and it felt as cleansing as the ray had been. I filled it with sweet smelling spring flowers and once again, my optimism grew.

A dream: A second meeting with the lion

I was driving along a country road. Lions were grazing in the open grassland. I was not afraid because I was in my car, but I knew if I had for some reason to open a door, or if for some reason a door flew open, I would be in danger.

I came to a bridge over a river. This part of the road was perilous. I needed to drive very carefully for there was little room. Somehow, although I did not plummet my car to the river below, the car tilted on the uneven narrow bridge and the doors flew open.

A great lion lumbered in where I was trapped. He bent over me and began gnawing away my left breast. As he ate I felt his flaccid, animal phallus brush against my leg.

14. Information from where?

"What does that make you think of?"

"I don't know! I just know that I feel very odd, quite strange."

"Well, tell me how you are feeling."

"I can see something but it doesn't make sense."

"We are not working with what makes sense. We are not working with what is logical. Just tell me what you see. Anything. Unusual or surprising. Tell me how you feel."

"Well . . . I can see myself standing on bare floorboards and I'm only dressed in a petticoat. All I can see is this white fog and then I seem to be standing quite still and my flesh is changing colour."

"Yes, go on."

I really struggle with the image because it feels as though I'm looking at myself from some strange vantage point that I've never experienced before. My flesh looks pink and young and full . . . now it's turning to a sort of a bluish tinged colour and . . . now it looks the colour of putty . . . and the white fog is thicker . . . and now it seems as though I'm outside my body and looking down and my body is on the floor.

My heart is racing and as I speak I almost feel as though I'm outside my body right now. The room has receded, everything around me seems to have gone away and nothing exists but Peter's voice and my own. I am frightened, very frightened and I feel as though if I were to lose touch with Peter's voice I would die. That sounds dramatic and maybe silly but that's how suddenly the room had altered from being an ordinary study to being a whole field of feelings and knowledge that had been hidden that I did not even know existed. "I feel terrible," I said "I feel frightened".

"You're all right," he said. "If you can just keep going."

"Now, it seems," I said, "that my body is just slowly disintegrating and all I can see is the petticoat lying on the floor, crumpled, and there are stains on the floor and then there is only dust."

"Where are you?"

"Here. I'm in this white fog and now I can't see anything and I'm very frightened."

"What else do you feel."

"I feel I don't know where I am. I don't know where I've been. I don't know where I'm going. I don't know where I am. I feel as though I'm a long way off." My heart still is beating wildly and my skin feels cold and clammy. "I feel disengaged from everything about me and then when the feeling is almost unbearable, when I think that I'll have to stop, hands come towards me taking me by the arm and leading me away. I can't see them, they too seem to have become formless, parts of the fog as I have become. But I can experience the sense of them taking me away. I can't see any more. That's all I can do for this session."

Still the feeling of the experience remains and I take some Bach rescue remedy from my bag and Peter gives me a glass of water. Slowly, while he speaks to me reassuringly, the feeling recedes, the white fog dissipates and I'm truly back in the room. I don't even think about what it means, I can't. It's just so strange and so odd. Often when very important things have come to me I've simply rested in a blankness as though I'm energizing myself again, until my mind can gather itself up to help to make sense of what has happened. Peter and I discuss it a little. We had been discussing a very ordinary, or what I had thought had been a very ordinary dream, and here out of the blue, as though impelled by other hands, I had gone in a different direction and discovered a landscape, a place and some knowledge that was totally unexpected. Like a traveller who has lost her way I had found a place that was not on the map. As Peter quietly and gently pointed out, what I had described was my own death and my passing out of my body. How could I describe my own death? I had experienced it as a thing of the past, not of the future. How had I done that? We were only at the first layer.

I went home bemused, bewildered and strangely excited. Frightened too, for there was still a lot that was unknown. I would need courage to go back to that place to explore it to look at the details, to wonder where the place was. This was work for the next session.

"How do you feel about last week?"

"I feel very strange and quite anxious."

"That's not surprising," he said. "You've had a most unusual experience. Have you thought more of what it means?"

"No I haven't. I feel that I don't know enough to come to any conclusions."

"Are you willing to go further with what you've seen?"

"Yes, I am," I said tentatively. "But I don't feel very brave about it."

"Well just remember that you can stop at any stage. Just say and you can stop. What happened last week is quite different from anything you've experienced before. Have you thought about our method of working?"

"No," I said.

"Well, you've achieved something quite spontaneously which psychologists and patients can do together quite consciously with some techniques. What you have done is to tap actively into your unconscious memory. What you had is not a waking dream, but an actual memory."

We were both quiet. I felt as though my mind should almost explode with such a revelation. Perhaps I recounted this in a way that isn't quite correct. I remember at the time that this was not actually a statement. In effect Peter's whole assessment of the situation was a tentative exploration, a quiet framing of a picture into which I could draw firm lines where I could come to my own conclusions.

"Shall we try again?" he asked. "I think what we need to do, is to find out where you were, find out where you died."

Again my heart began to pound, and as I sat comfortably in the chair, feeling the strength of certainty that Peter had, I felt as though somebody had just walked in front of me and was standing by my shoulder.

"Peter", I said "I feel as though there is someone else in the room." I was quite certain there was.

"There is no one to be seen," he said, "but stranger things have happened. Perhaps someone is standing guard, someone is protecting you so that our explorations will be quite safe."

"Somebody from the spiritual world," I said to myself.

It wasn't the first time I'd experienced this sense of unseen presence. This tangible inner feeling as if you could see the form with your physical senses, and so I felt comforted. We began.

"Do you feel quite comfortable?"

"Yes," I said tremulously.

"Just relax and let yourself relax your mind and remember that this is not an academic logical experience belonging to the physical world. It's something else. So tell me everything you see and everything you feel no matter how silly or bizarre it seems."

15. The distant past

Why didn't anyone hear me? Why didn't they hear me?

It was such a beautiful day. The day was filled with yellow sunshine. It was the kind of day so dense with golden light, that if an apple fell from its tree, it would be suspended in the rich fecundity of the air. This day's events changed the direction of my destiny — such an event should not have happened on such a day.

It happened when I went looking for my child. She was a bright, intelligent two year old, with the prettiness of the young Goldilocks, who had never been walking in the woods. I can see us standing before the place — I had found my little one, playing there, picking wild flowers as yellow as the sun, quite oblivious of the moment. And so was I. There I was, the sleeves of my calico dress rolled up, bare legged, blossoming in full female beauty, knowing that I was loved, holding my daughter's hand, looking at a cellar door in the hillside.

I can see it as if in a tableau — suspended in time like the golden apples. I was all pale beige and beautiful, tall and full of the late summer light, holding the hand of my precious child who trailed a rag doll behind her, its long legs sprawling in the dust. I can see us like a framed photograph, facing the cellar door.

The place looked deserted. I was drawn to that door as surely as one of those apples inevitably is drawn to the ground. I opened the door. Sun fell in a long slice of light across a decaying wooden floor. I dropped my daughter's hand. As I hesitated on the doorstep I noticed kegs in the corner and the moving stain of dark red wine which flowed from one of the dusky shapes. "Go home," I whispered, turning in the doorway, seeing for the last time the clear blue eyes of my cherished child who was already turning for flight, hugging the much loved form of her lifeless toy, whose blank, embroidered eyes stare at me still.

At first there seemed to be nobody there, only a dark malevolence seemed to fill the gloom and then as my eyes accustomed themselves to the darkness and they lost the image of the sunlight, I saw a dark, short, stocky man standing quietly in the corner. He was carrying a horse-whip. He looked at me without speaking, holding me

*with his gaze. Stretched out before him, his whip lay
on the floor with the impression of being capable of
moving into dastardly life at any moment.*

*"And so you've come," he said. I just looked at him.
I knew who he was. I recognized him. Then in an
instant he sprang towards me, light on his feet and his
grasp of my arm was impossible to resist. He began to
kiss me, greedily and tauntingly. I lost my breath and
then I began to scream, I screamed as though my life
depended upon it. I screamed for my lover. No one
came. He growled and grunted like an animal. He was
angry, beyond himself, out of control. He ripped the
front of my calico shift and beneath it I was almost
bare. A simple chemise was all I wore; that too was
ripped from me. My struggles to free myself only gave
energy to the pulling and pushing, the ripping and
tearing of my clothing from me.*

*"Oh God," I cried, "Please God save me." But he
did not. With a great push and a slap as I screamed
even louder I was hurled to the floor. As I fell I lifted
my knees but his weight came down as if my bones were
breaking. And then he was upon me shifting and
heaving as if to kill me with his presence. My screaming
turned to anguished crying, sobbing that took all my
breath away and as he jerked and pushed almost muti-
lating my inside as well as bruising my outside, I felt
that I would die from shame. This was mortification
indeed. As he flung the last angry, hot lash of himself
into me I thought I'd die. I felt spent. As though the
fury of his assault had caught me like ropes and pulled
me in. I was like an animal in a trap. A rabbit with
its foot caught, waiting to have its neck broken, waiting
for death.*

And then I gathered myself together, but instead of a

*scream for help — I was sick. The smell of his flesh
and his coming blended with my vomit. Again my
vomiting had brought him back to action. For me to be
sick at his act made him terrifyingly angry. He swore
at me over and over, and from his belt he drew a knife
and with words that I'd never heard before he cut into
my breast, slashing through it as if to part my being.
The look on my face, the life that still remained there
seemed to egg him on in a fury. The disgust and all my
feelings that rose to face him in my eyes drove him
further. The knife came down and slashed my face. It
came across my eyes and as it did so the pain was white
hot. Blood-warm, sweet, rich, red blood flowed from
my eyes and my face and my breast and I knew I would
die.*

*I was beyond screams, I was beyond the anguish of
crying or even moaning. The feeling of that assault, the
strength of the hate that had lived in him seemed to enter
my soul. It overcame me as surely as if I was strangled.
I felt my life streaming from me as the blood flowed in
a river to join the spilt red wine on the dusty floor. And
then feelings of grief, overwhelming grief, tears, unshed,
filled my inner being until I was drowned in them. And
then I was nothing but feeling. And my feeling seemed
to flow out and about me, I was bodyless, empty. My
life had been shed. Thankfully the pain, the dreadful
pain, was gone. Death had brought me escape. He could
touch me no longer. The grief receded. There was no
feeling. I was just me. Nobody. Feeling no past, no
future, and the hands that led me away from the place,
laid me down to be healed. None of this could be
seen or felt in the ordinary way. It was something that
happened. My whole body was bandaged in strands of
light. Fingers moved across my wounds, and as they did*

I felt whole again. Forming light drew my body together like a weaving and as each finger stroke mended me a sound arose, a chord that was one sound which swelled and radiated like the ripples of a stone plunged into a pool. Further and further the sound radiated but did not fade as ripples disperse. It simply became richer, more profound, more lasting, and it was as if the light and the sound became one and a thousand voices carried the sound and reformed my body. I was uplifted, sustained and myself again; safe, perfect, and at rest.

The night I recounted this experience to Peter I was devastated. All the feelings of the experience flooded into me and were as real as if I were experiencing it again. I've never cried as I cried that night. I was awash with the anguish, with the grief, with the mortification, and then there was the promise of peace.

For the following week I was shocked, I was deeply shocked. I knew that this retelling was indeed a retelling. It was not fantasy, it was an all-encompassing happening. It could not be anything else but memory and so for the first time in my own experience the thought of having lived before came to me as a real possibility. Actually I was not interested in forming theories, I was only interested in making sense of my own destiny. In an effort to expunge the terrible nature of that death, I retold this experience for several weeks until I could do so without tears and without destructive feeling. As I did this it seemed to me that darkened corners were being brought into the light and that I was then cleansed.

In our working together it came to both Peter and

me that in fact I was re-enacting all the terrible, shocking, sudden aspects of that untimely death in this life. The loss of breath with my asthma, the loss of my breast, blindness, cuts on my face and, although I did not know it, in the future the pain of bones almost breaking apart. What this meant perhaps was that in the ingesting, the working through of all these aspects had not been possible because of the sudden nature of my former death. So in this lifetime each one of them had to be met, experienced and consciously worked through so that the person, the individual ego that was me could shed them like outer layers of clothing. It came to me, not then, but a long way in the future, that each life has aspects of experience like this; that each life is like a set of clothing which becomes besmirched, tattered, rent, showing signs of all these experiences and as the outer clothing, that is the body, is deteriorated by its experience, death comes as a salve to cleanse, to purify and to spiritualize what has happened in our earthly life.

At that time I did not understand it all, but I knew that for the first time in therapy we were getting to the guts of the problem, we were forming a structure, a grid from which to weave the rebuilding of myself. I was deeply thankful for the fact that Peter, as a counsellor, was not enslaved by a rigid doctrine of this or that particular therapy. He was open and sensitive to what was real and what was delusion. As we sat together working through what was a most crucial turning point in my life, I felt his cool scrutiny of my whole situation as a taut strong thread. He was supporting me in a way that I knew was crystal clear, disinterested, but infused with a feeling for human life and human endeavour that was rare. I was to learn in the future that his knowledge of Christ was not a fairy-book image which he wore in front of him, but this knowledge of Christ penetrated everything that he thought and did. He was not a Bible basher, a born-again Christian, he was a person in contact with a force that was, in essence, Love.

This experience of Peter as a stable rudder in all my searching did not come at once, but unfolded before me in the same way as the meaning of my life unfolded.

A dream: A third meeting with the lion

A young child stood at my skirts. Together we viewed lions moving about in a grassy paddock. I was afraid, but she was unperturbed knowing that we were simply aware of each other — in truce you might say.

16. A critical reverie and meditation

What can I see in my minds eye? What can I see in the past? I can only see what was in my field of vision if I were standing, but I am not standing — I am kneeling — with my breasts on my knees, with my arms tucked in as if to protect myself. I feel very young and strong inside. I have a strong body . . . a young woman's body. As I kneel there, I feel the strength of real knowledge within me . . . knowledge that I cannot tell anyone, and yet I know that others know.

I can see the deep wool carpet a few inches from my face. It is a deep emerald green, the green that is in the heart of grass on a full summer's day when it is at the height of its growth, past its pale and tender age. It is full and deep and rich. It is the kind of green that has blue hidden in its centre. It is not the overgrown green of the forest where leaves grow dark and mysterious. It has no lustre. It has no edge. It is full.

On my left there is a large glass cabinet, full of precious things, with tiny glass segments like those in the french doors. Beside the doors are velvet drapes to pull at night, to keep the privacy of the room, its warmth and its memorable splendour. They are not emerald green. I can't see what colour they are. And yet I know they are a nuance of the same melody.

And outside it is full summer. There is no damp . . . there is full dry sunshine. Someone outside is listening, someone who knows my secret is listening just beyond the french doors. I've seen his face before. I have seen it appear in my blank vision, in the veil that is before my eyes. His face appeared first as the face of a small laughing child, a mischievous child. Those eyes were bright lustrous pale blue . . . shining blue like glass. Then his smiling face changed to that of an adult lout — one who taunts, one who terrifies young women, for all he has is his physical strength . . . his animal overpowering strength. He creates fear and yet, like a tiger, he does not come into the open. He is not the lion of my dreams. He is the hidden tiger, camouflaged in my deepest knowledge.

Now, before me I can see the riding boots, dusty . . . dusty. And their angle shows fear too, of unacknowledged truth. The tail of the whip lies coiled but with the air of a flaccid phallus, upon the carpet. It is as though it is sleeping, waiting for its owner to wield when sureness returns. I cannot see his face but he is young, very young. He is a master and he is jealous.

In the corner of the room, the right hand corner, beside the velvet drape which seems now to have an olive curve on the fold, is a simple circular table — it shines and is reflecting the contents of the room. It has a long central pedestal which flows down to the floor into four feet and above them, almost to the ground, is a small circle of timber which echoes the top of the table. I've never seen a table like this.

I've told Peter that I know that my inheritance is this house. My father lives here, yet my plaited braids, my apron, my bare arms and feet seem still to be covered with the light of outside — I work for this house. I have been displaced . . . yet my inheritance is a deep loving memory. My young blood and my young passion can be expressed in the simple ways of the people I live with. If I love, I can show that I love, if I hate, I can spit and claw — I am a passionate creature.

I feel that in the future, perhaps in another life, I will know the gentler ways of those who love books and who arrange flowers in the way they are arranged on the table here in this room. They stand, arranged, fully prepared for appraisal in an oriental vase with many sides.

It is blue . . . oriental blue . . . . . . and now I remember the healing . . . my spiritual healer whom I have never met till now. I can see him, his long white hair and his round spectacles and his laughing tender face. He is wise. He has been my teacher. He is still my teacher. Marlene has spoken with him but I have not even glimpsed him until now.

Through my streaming memories, the strands of my inheritance, my spiritual inheritance, are floating in a pool, moving quietly. Soon I will see them all . . . and when at last I see them, they will become like beds of rock. Then the water, the moving clear water, the living spring, will be truly clear and transparent, glowing and cool . . . a mirror . . . transformed white light. A mirror. Then . . . I will SEE. . . .

The black crows will return to the dead trees. I'll not see them fly through the living. The currawong in its ease and strong casual beauty unnoticed, will join the city with the open country that I love, so that my being will be everywhere with the currawong.

I turned over in my bed to relive this meditation consciously. I have listened to the words and now I know the truth . . . and I don't like it. It's gone like a sword into my stomach. As I lay listening to the words again, reading what I had written, in consciousness, listening to the words, I saw that young man and I knew that he was my brother. I knew that it was he who had lain in wait. He killed me. That flaccid whip on the floor became the degrading instrument which lay with me in death. But he was not truly my brother. He was half my brother, my half-brother. His blackness did not come from our father. He knew not my mother.

I wondered what had called me to that place. It was not the sweet smell of love, it was not the invitation to a liaison. It was the call of blood, of half my blood. It had run in the wrong direction. My brother, who was not my brother. I was not destroyed by the physical power of death, but I was mauled and beaten; an incestuous degradation.

Filial love I didn't know. My father, I've not yet known my father.

Black nature — a black garb? Perhaps it was his riding suit. I don't know which garb he wore. Perhaps it was his nature on his sleeve. Perhaps the four black buttons were like four black crows, close to the dying.

How can I carry this truth? How can I take the veil from the bright day. My teacher, my beloved partner in life, my lost child, my father. Where are they? Where are the hands that guided me to rest and restoration? I want not just my teacher, I want love. I want the truth to be love. And love to be truth. I need life to caress me . . . and say that I am loved . . . that I am worthy. I want my child in easy knowledge.

I am with God but I want to be with the earth; not with the dust but in the living clay. I want to be a round, warm loving wife, a partner, a mate. I want the rose within me to grow to answer the call of the sun. I want to unfold into full bloom.

I want to be cleansed. Is the message of the Christ related? My feeling is frozen, locked still in the place from where my knowledge has sprung. I must be warmed, I must be safe, to let it free. Perhaps my tears are the cool, clear pool.

Where is irrepressible, unconscious joy? That is what I want. Not this intense, conscious, drawing of the sword from my soul.

17. Growing in new directions

In the following months I began taking Iscador, a live substance of mistletoe, which by nature is very like cancer. It is a homoeopathic remedy but is used by some orthodox doctors as an ordinary drug. It increases the white blood cell activity, stimulates the immune system and helps to increase body warmth. It is therefore given early in the morning to catch the tide of the rising body temperature which reaches its peak at about five in the afternoon. I'd been wanting to take this remedy, or to have this remedy as an injection, for quite some time, but a series of slip-ups had made it impossible. About a fortnight after I had been having the injections I discovered another lump in the area where my left breast had been. I was shaken by this discovery for I'd had a great deal of confidence in the Iscador. And of course it was still only five months since I'd had the ray treatment. I thought quickly and acted promptly. I decided that if the Iscador was to help I'd have to find out more about it and that the only place to find out about it was to go to the London Homoeopathic Hospital, to the Cancer Clinic, where I could consult with Dr Twentyman, who was in charge of that Clinic. He had prescribed the Iscador for me through a local doctor who'd known him in London during her years of training. We made the arrangements and in a great hurry I rang Joan early one morning and asked her, if we were to help with the fare, would she be able to accompany me for the three-week stay in London. In Joan's usual direct style, she said "Yes" and in ten days we were on the plane flying to London.

Within the course of a few months my life had changed from a very ordinary suburban one on the outside to a complex new kind of life which was opening up within me. I had found the events which materialized in therapy at first almost unbelievable, and then I had found difficulty in asking a friend who was a nurse to give me this homoeopathic remedy for cancer. I was afraid she would think I was silly, some kind of nut, but she didn't. I explained to her that I would not have chemotherapy. The specialist who had ordered my ray treatment had, when I revisited him with this lump, suggested that I have six months of chemo-therapy and have my ovaries removed. I couldn't accept either of those suggestions. This may not have been an entirely logical decision, but every part of me was repulsed by the idea and rejected it. Somehow if I were to achieve health in my lifetime it had to be worked through consciously; that is, what came to me had to be worked through consciously, and I had decided that not another part of my body was going to be lopped off. I felt that the shock, the destructive shock, of having more surgery after all the anaesthetics and surgery I'd already had (almost a dozen) my natural resources would be impaired beyond what was reasonable. I also felt that the chemo-therapy would do the same thing.

Dr Twentyman's surgery was as little like a doctor's surgery as I could imagine. It had a most serene atmosphere, I sat on a brocade couch which he told me was decorated with Indian elephants doing all sorts of marvellous things. A small table with a bowl of water was by our side, and English early spring flowers floated on the surface of the water. He sat almost next to me in a comfortable chair and so began a short but most intense and serious meeting. I saw him three times; each time we covered as much ground as you would normally expect in weeks or months. Our exchanges were distilled to such a point that I was able afterwards to fill out the ideas which we had talked of in essence. Dr Twentyman answered my lists of questions with patience and a great deal of detail.

Joan had decided that she couldn't possibly give me my injections every second day, but when I related this to Dr Twentyman he took things in his own hands and before she knew it, there was Joan being given a lesson, and Dr Twentyman in a short time demystified the whole thing of giving injections.

We had set ourselves up in a very cheap, sleazy

flat that we would come home to in the afternoons. While I slept for four or five hours Joan would read, lying on the floor at my feet, for there was little else to do, and at about nine-thirty she would make a simple meal with the limited equipment we had, and finally at about ten-thirty we would both go to sleep. Almost every night she read for at least half an hour. I would sometimes say "Joan, you've been doing things for me all day, don't you want some time to yourself?"

"No" she'd say. "Do you want to read or don't you?" and so we would.

She organized, as a special surprise for me, a visit to the Tate Gallery. She refused to tell me that morning where we were going but as we trundled up out of the underground I happened to recognize something of the spatial landscape perceptible to me, and I commented that we'd been there just a few days previously. The exhibition I was shown (I had a private showing) was a retrospective exhibition of British sculpture which had come home from all over the world. Among the pieces that had fallen and broken at the Museum of Modern Art, pieces from the Guggenheim, from all over Europe, there I was with Joan and the Curator, keeping an ear out for any important personages who might exclaim that I shouldn't be touching all the pieces. I saw the most exquisite Barbara Hepworth basalt sculpture in which a small leaf was embedded and fossilized. I could readily place it in the southern landscape of England which we had visited the previous week. In fact as my hands moved over the various pieces, especially the Henry Moores, I had exactly the same feeling as I'd had when I could see, standing on the crest of a hill or in some place that could be considered a lookout. As my eyes had previously travelled over the curves, crevices, the rhythmical folding and unfolding of the earth's surface, now my hands moved as though in the same essential stream of movement that had created the hills and the valleys. This was food for my soul that I had been deprived of for years. I'd spent many happy hours in museums and art galleries filling myself with the essential truth that the artist captures. Each artist seems to get a glimmer or a fragment of what I'm sure we will only understand after death.

When I left that gallery my hands were absolutely black from all the dust, for the exhibition was yet to be opened by Queen Elizabeth. I didn't simply feel pleasure at having had a preview of a very important Exhibition. I felt that I'd been in touch with a part of myself, with a communicating part of myself, a passageway that had been closed, blocked off for some time. I had exactly the same feeling when we visited the south of England. We hired a car, and each day we would travel a certain distance, stopping, just here and there, sometimes simply to walk by the side of the road, to clamber over fences, to sit under trees, to investigate small village churches, and so on.

When we went into Chichester Cathedral the first Sunday and I heard the rising, echoing voices of a large, well-practised choir, I felt supported, and when I heard the sermon of the resurrection from the Letters to the Corinthians, every word seemed to have been spoken just for me. The possibility of early death was now real. The Iscador could help, but could I expect a cure? In the following days we were very appreciative tourists and my visit to Winchester Cathedral was like a coming home. Had I really been there before? Had my consciousness, in a different body, walked in that place before? The whole building seemed to be alive with the weaving, moving consciousness of the hundreds of people who had walked on those flagstone floors. Every memorial tablet, every step, every stepping stone seemed to stand in place of someone who had known the Cathedral. It seemed as though suddenly time was not important and I was walking with the multitude.

When I got to the border of Dorset and Cornwall I actually felt as though I was home. The landscape was utterly familiar and in one section where we drove off the main roads I felt as though we had found a valley, a place where I might have lived in that former life. In the rugged terrain of this area, people had stored their smuggled wine and spirits in hillside cellars. This knowledge came to me while I was there and just as I had been drawn into that cellar in that past life, I'd now been drawn to the south of England to travel a road that I almost knew.

We went to Tintagel at the end of the day, and this too had the same feeling as Winchester Cathedral: as though it were peopled again by thousands, silent, but their presences about me. And when we reached the top of the hill where part of the castle still stood Joan tried to take a photograph across the chasm of the piece that had broken away, but King Arthur's seat was not to be photographed. The sun was at such an angle that its brilliance filled the area with blinding golden light. To my perceptions it seemed to be a mirror and this in a way is what my whole visit to England was. A kind of mirror image of what actually was inside me, but which I'd not previously been able to see.

"Mummy," I cried as I jumped off my bike throwing it against the front fence and confronting my mother almost in the same movement and the same breath. "Judy Orth says there's no Father Christmas — there is, isn't there?" I was scandalized, horrified and very earnest.

"Oh, yes," my mother said, transferring sewing pins from her mouth to the saucer beside her. "Oh yes," she said, resuming her stitching in easy predictable movements. "He is the spirit of Christmas."

"I knew he was," I said with satisfaction. And I did know, for I was eight years old, no longer a beginner in life who only knows the literal truth.

As the years have gone by I have often thought about the anonymous, mysterious giving which parents indulge in for their youngsters in their celebration of the birth of Christ.

On our trip to Winchester Cathedral I learnt more about the English Saint Nicholas — one of the inspirations for our symbolic giving to children at Christmas. Joan, my travelling companion, went 'shutter-bugging' the wonders we had already seen in our tour of the ancient cathedral. During my quiet meditation in a side aisle, I heard enough of a story of the font nearby from a tourist guide to suggest to Joan on her return that we should have a closer inspection of this memorial to St Nicholas. My fingers were travelling in the rather crude but beautiful bas-relief of that font, when a strong, elderly voice asked if I knew anything about the saint. Miss Purdy, proclaimed as 'volunteer guide' by the notice on her lapel, was quite an ambassador for the friends of the cathedral group. She was over seventy and as lively and dedicated as the atmosphere of the cathedral.

The font was carved from black basalt in the tenth century depicting all the stories of Bishop Nicholas, as he was then, and the happy endings. Among the four tales on the sides of the font, one depicts Bishop Nicholas saving two young men from the butcher's knife being wielded by an inn-keeper who had decided to convert the two youths into sausage-mince to feed some unsuspecting, rich travellers. (Could this story have inspired the saying, 'in the nick of time'?)

Two young boys from St Nicholas' College didn't know what the three bags of gold on their black blazer pocket meant. Miss Purdy told us of the origin of that emblem, pointing to another story. Apparently three village maids were in disgrace because they had no dowry. Consequently no suitors were at hand. Bishop Nicholas heard of their plight and supplied each with their own bag of gold, and of course everyone got their just deserts . . . including the Bishop who was later canonized.

Some of my ancestors could have worshipped here. What gifts we have in re-living the past. All those links in the chain seem to form frames in which there is a face, a story, a relationship with the form of our lives today.

As we climbed the pilgrim steps from the original parish church, I thought of my own dead father who lies buried in foreign soil. My own personal loss fell from me like a discarded cloak, to lie amongst the shadows of the past. His spirit seemed to join the army of dead souls who had become symbols of sacrifice. The words of the present minister filled my ears. "Several times a day we pause together to remember that this ancient Cathedral is a house of God and a place of worship and prayer . . . Our Father . . . and may the peace of God go in your hearts . . . "

I stepped out of the church into the pale golden light of English spring sunshine, as pale and as fragile as the first daffodils by the side of the path.

Father Christmas, loving tributes in stone, the gift of life in every new generation, and every new spring. . . . every step on that cobblestoned path gave way to pulsing thoughts moving into another corner of my mind. My feet were in the past for we are as Lord Tennyson has said "a part of all that we have met".

Inside that ancient church, the sun had thrown facets of stained light on the shoulders of the congregation, through the giant rose window of the altar. Now the sun shone on my face while new thoughts and connecting ideas sprang to life within me, moving like great coloured pieces of a kaleidoscope. Soon they would come to rest, forming new patterns which would create new directions for my life.

As an adult I know that Father Christmas is only a symbol of the spirit of Christmas; I know what the spirit of Christmas really means. I also know that Winchester Cathedral, built in 1078, is one of the glorious manifestations of the spiritual journey which centuries of pilgrims are inspired to make.

Every day from the time we left the south of England I longed to be home. I missed Ben and Kate as a body misses its limbs, and as I sat in the plane, distraught with fatigue and feeling assaulted by the artificial atmosphere, I was kept alive in my optimism by the thought of the quality of the air that would greet me when I got out of the car at our front gate. I knew that it would be cool, with autumn coolness, I knew that it would be fresh and revitalized by the trees and that all the strong life of our garden and the living smell of our wooden house would greet me and fill me up again. I knew that Ben's strong arms and warm breath would fill me out again and that Kate's little hand would once more be in mine.

18. Home again. Winter, June 1978

I've never felt so alive as I did that morning. I began to wake very early. I listened to the birds' sound — like messengers for the morning — one here, one there, filling in the dimness of space outside my window. I could tell it would be one of those perfect days that has the quality of season changing from winter to spring or summer to autumn. I wonder if I woke from a long coma, if I would know which it was without looking at the quality and colour of the leaves.

As I lay there, feeling every sense fill my being with acute stinging warmth, and rising to know every bit of it with the clarity that dreadful shock gives us. A tiny sound of small feet on the carpet . . . I pushed aside the blankets. Katie crawled in beside me, tucking her bottom into my stomach and her head pressed next to mine on the pillow. Ben was curled against my back, our warmth mingling, enclosed in blankets and bed. The scattered spots of sound were drawn together as a light plane mechanically droned its way across the sky above our heads.

"Mummy", Katie whispered, "I think that's a jumbo jet."

A friend had been talking about her own daughter flying off to England in a jumbo the night before.

"Not quite, darling," I said. "It's just one of those little planes that fly over nearly every day."

"I think," she said, disturbing the cave; concaving the line of the blankets as she rose up, disturbing our drowsy position, "little planes should be just for little children, middle sized planes for mummies and jumbo jets for dads."

"Do you?" I said, noncommittal, vaguely aware of this modern version of Goldilocks. I turned hugging Ben and his warmth to me knowing that I must respond to the "Mummy, please get my breakfast".

It was Sunday morning when the world could be our bed; just the three of us, playing games of "I spy", telling desultory stories based on our past, hugging in pairs and together, making patterns with our legs, our arms, and all of us beneath the covers.

Later I made tea, took it back to bed where Ben and I made love and I mean made love. It was that seeking to be one, that driving need never to be parted. I loved like my first love. Without reason, but for all reasons, in absolute trust, as though we know each other — there is no revelation of two ego beings — we came together and we come together — our bodies fell apart, we drifted without consultation into conversation about our future. What would Katie do, who would be her guardian? It is useless, our sacred trust of parenthood cannot be carried out by anyone else. Who else will hold her in their arms in the way I do? Who else will glory in her as she will be? I have seen who she is and who she must be. Who else will guard her, shield her and love her for her Katieness? Why do I feel that Ben and I will never be parted, even by death, while I cannot face that separation from the being who came to us through birth, a part of our flesh and out of our union?

How can a mother relinquish her cherished trust? I cannot bear to leave the gift to earth, who came through me and to me.

I said to Ben, "Every time a child is born to us, we have the chance to make the earth a better place, by making sure our children grow to be what they themselves are, each and every one a unique gift to earth in our lifetime."

I lie in bed by myself. Ben sings in the shower and I think about my death dispassionately, listening to Katie's return with her playmate, my mind in focus, as my tears stream inward. I am here, today I am here. Will I feel so acutely alive every day I am here!

The whole family woke early this Sunday morning when we could easily have had a beautiful sleep-in.

I heard Katie get up and put on her light. Of course she made straight for the television. She has only just discovered the commercial stations, with all their fascination of the market place and the amoral flavour of advertisement after advertisement.

I wonder if I let her make a glutton of herself? Will she get sick of it all and be more discriminating? Tiny predigested vignettes from all over the world, passing straight into the ingenuous vision of a six-year-old seems to me to be pretty dangerous medicine. A friend's sister plied her four-year-old with copious amounts of chocolate until he voluntarily said 'no' to the supply that was available. It might have had a permanent effect on his appetite for chocolate, but what if there was permanent damage to who knows what? I've limited television watching for Kate so far. I wonder if it's safe now for her to take some of that responsibility herself?

When the light first went on, I was sure it was only just getting light. It's truly winter. The darkness lets go its grip unwillingly. The birds are desultory in their revels. It has been raining in soft spasms for several days. I used to hate the winter, but at present it suits my mood. It's good to be inside, safe and uncommitted. The day has less form, so thoughts drift in and out with my slowly unfolding activities. The rain is slightly melancholy, but gently so. It has no despairing turbulence. It seems to be quietly, persistently soaking the dead leaves of autumn into the ground, and softening the hard unyielding areas of clay that were thrown up when the foundations of our new house were being built last year. We seem to have come a long way. I know that we will eventually tame our garden, if we can co-operate

143

with it so that its growth can go on in harmony with our needs. The flowers and all the growth beneath the sentinel trees will come together, framing the house, our house, in easy beauty.

Winter. Like the bears and snakes all over the world, I hibernated. I had a strict routine where I had a lot of sleep, I meditated at least three times a day and on several occasions I had sessions of deep relaxation. In between I really entered with great pleasure into the structuring of each day. Sometimes I would get up in the morning and feel a lack of strength, but as I began to work quietly into the day, doing daily chores, housework, I found that I was building my strength. As well as this very strong structure I still had a need for creative work and it was during this time I did quite a lot of writing. It was a time of quiet pleasure. From time to time I looked at the lump on my chest, but then I decided that seeing it didn't seem to be doing much, I should just try and ignore it and go about my business, go about my living. I began eurythmy, which is a really involving form of rhythmical movement, descriptive movement. I was quite surprised that I managed to move about with a group of up to twelve people and stay within the forms we created, most of the time. And if I was given time to develop and experience the form I could do it as well as the rest.

I had for so many years lived completely in the outside world, dependent on other people or perhaps not so much dependent but very interested and involved with other people and projects. I'd had a very lively political life, and now I had to give up all of this life outside me.

144

In a way it was giving up life, that is how I felt about it first, then of course one of the saints said that we must die in order to live again. It was very hard to let go of the work which expressed my personality and which gave me a sense of worth in an outside way. I gave up editing a magazine for blind people which I'd begun; I stopped working for the Braille Library for the time being, although I didn't officially resign; and I stopped speaking to various groups and being involved in all the multitudinous activities which had come my way in the past. This could be anything from speaking to architecture students on architecture and what it means for a person without sight, to speaking very personally about my own life and how the various experiences had changed and altered me, or again speaking with student nurses about the needs of visually handicapped people in hospital.

From that activity I went to this quiet period of time when nearly all of my activity was either inward or simply physical.

Meditation had become a working and an experiencing which grew more important to me. That winter of hibernation was truly a sleep, a rest from the turmoil and difficulties of the outer world, a time for my body to rest in the support of its very tentative spiritual growth and a time for me to look at my self. Not in a searching way, not in a really heady kind of way, but simply a quiet objective appraisal. In late July I thought that the lump was slightly smaller, but I didn't say anything to anyone, just allowing it to remain in a corner of my consciousness. And then one day I couldn't find it. I began to swim in a bath of warm joy. I made an appointment with the doctor and suggested she might like to look and see how it was going. I was like a child with a most beautiful parcel which I was wanting to share, and I wanted her to have the same sense of surprise as I had had. There was definitely no lump there, I was free of it. I came out as the flowers came out in the spring. I had three articles published in *The Age*, I appeared on two television shows speaking about my experiences and within a couple of months I was in full swing again. What foolishness that was! And yet life kept drawing me into its orbit in a way that made me want to draw back, to keep the balance between the outer and the inner, and this has been a constant, most difficult thing to achieve.

In the meantime I felt reprieved and I hardly dared to whisper to myself that there was a possibility that I could once again get better. Peter kept reminding me that I had to realize that even though the cancer was now not overt there was a real possibility of its appearing again and that for some time I had to treat myself with great care. I listened and I saw the sense of it, but I found it impossible to do. Life was too strong in its call for vigorous, whole-hearted involvement.

My period. Today when I was changing, I could smell my warm, fresh blood and I realized, truly (not as it is when you have a passing thought or an idea which you just put on for size), I realized that the flow from my nest would soon diminish until finally it would be no more. The fertile period of my life would be over. There would be no more babies from my being; I would not cradle another baby of my own in my arms; I could not croon it to sleep, passing it over into its bed, watching it in sleep, feeling the first sense of loss, giving it the warmth of my thoughts and remembering the giving of my life's blood from my breasts, and blessing the manner of its creation.

I knew when my breast was taken that I would not have another child. But at least then I could still have my dreams; my fantasies of how other mastectomies had had children, of supposing what it would be like if I suddenly knew that I was healed, irrevocably healed. But soon I will be unable to choose, in waking wisdom or in foolish dream.

Menopause. What an ugly word. How can I be hopeful about a new or a change of life when I have not fully experienced the last one? Every woman seems to have the capacity to carry, and nurture a certain number of offspring. My brood is not complete in size or in fruition. I was not ready for some who had chosen to come to earth by my side. I rejected others and one I left behind. Forgive me children, for I grieve for you now. The only child I have is now more precious than I can bear. Now, when I should almost be grandmothering, I see my future stretching before me in endless fear for my only child. Can I stay with her, strong and in touch with today? Already I have lived more than several lifetimes during this stay on earth. I need new strength . . . I need new light. I need the pulse in the ground to pump new red in my veins, to bring back warmth to my heart.

A dream: The last meeting with the lion

I was crouched low against a small outcrop of rock. Above me a hunter lay in a cave with a shotgun and wearing a pith helmet. A lion appeared, crouched, then sprang towards me. I willed the hunter to save me. His gun was pointed over my shoulder. He fired and the lion fell dead at my feet.

19. My mother's death

All day I had felt frail, not in charge of myself, unable to make a decision, kind of bloodless and depressed. Early in the morning I had been unable to gather Katie up in the energy which would take her to school. She wanted to stay home; she seemed to want just to stay close by me. I'd already made arrangements to see Liz during the morning, so the only thing I managed to do was to breakfast Kate and me, dress us, and arrive on her doorstep. I spent the morning in desultory conversation, having numerous cups of tea, and in early afternoon I knew that I should go home to rest. But there was a vague uneasiness about going home. There had been a rapist at large in our area, and I loathed the idea of going into an empty house. If I stayed, Graeme would take me home later in the day. The whole complexity of making a decision was just too much for me, so I just sat on, knowing that I was getting more and more tired and that that evening I had eurythmy. Eurythmy required a lot of physical presence and, this I did not have. During eurythmy, after the first feeble effort to participate, I sat on the floor, on the fringe, feeling a little strength from just being there where people were working in a strong individual manner and contributing to the group.

It was with absolute relief that I climbed into bed and pulled the warm blankets up over my shoulders. It was Friday, October the 5th, the day before Cheryl's birthday. I lay in bed feeling the shape of my body beneath the blankets and waiting for warmth and strength to return. I had a sense of disquiet and before this was truly formed, the phone jangled into it. There, as I picked up the receiver, was Di ringing from Mount Gambier.

"Hullo Max. Is Ben there?"

"Yes he is, but what's the matter? Won't I do?"

Silence, then, "I'd like to speak to Ben."

"You can tell me. What is it? Is it Mum?"

"Yes . . . it's awful."

"The worst? Is she dead?"

"Yes. Dad found her tonight. We don't know how long she has been dead. He left on Wednesday for work and tonight, when he returned, there were no lights, no fire and nothing had been shifted. She's obviously collapsed."

I asked her question after question but she knew no more, or she would not say. I said I'd ring later when Father had settled down and had been able to tell the story. Actually it was no use, I was not to learn the true details until I got to Mount Gambier.

I cried for the death of my mother and for the absolute waste of all those painful years when she'd been waiting for death. How long had she been in the house, maybe still alive, not being able to get help? Had she wanted me? Had she wanted to join my own father? Had she thought of my stepfather as she was leaving? Had her death been sudden, without pain, with hardly a thought for the living? Every inch of me sensed that in the end she'd left reluctantly, that all that day she had been pulling at my strength, at my love for her and that she had tried to cling to life. I could feel no more and think no more. I left Ben's comforting arms and slipped beneath the blankets to rest. I prayed for her briefly and then for several peaceful hours I slept.

In the early hours of the morning I was woken by somebody calling. I did not hear my name, nor "Mummy", but I woke thinking it was Kate. I listened; there was not a sound. If Kate was fast asleep, it must be my mother, I thought, she still wants something from me. I prayed for her again, and then tried to sleep once more, for all the exhaustion of my feelings for my mother and the support I tried to give her, seemed to lie on me year upon year upon year. All I wanted to do was sleep. Just as I seemed to be dozing off, the bed started to shake violently. I woke again to find that it was really quite still; it was physically quite still. My mother, I thought again. She needs me. I rolled on to my back, several cushions beneath my head, I meditated long and fully, with absolute concentration, I imagined her body lying in death. I imagined the spiritual helpers waiting for her, taking her by her hands, soothing her, releasing the pain and giving her healing. I was thankful for my own experience of my past death, for in this way I could actually imagine what was happening.

I prayed for the love and support of thoughts from other people who knew her, and I asked heaven to cradle her until she had passed fully into the spiritual world. In asking for other people's thoughts, I began to think of Cheryl. It was already her birthday. She was the child who had been so bruised, actually damaged by my mother's illness. She'd always said that she didn't love my mother as much as her father. Somehow or other, she gave up a part of our mother to Brett, Graeme and to me. But her father, she kept all to herself. Sometimes she said she hated our mother. I knew this hatred was a hatred of the disease and that the anger and bitterness against our mother was Cheryl's inability to see the disease as something quite apart from the relationship she had with each of us, including her father. I wondered how we could blot out the sense of my mother as the person that she had become when she was ill. How could I restore to my family's memory the essential person that my mother had been in the beginning. That gay, optimistic, talented, energetic, free spirit. Cheryl would have been proud of her if she had known her in those early days.

In the past years my mother's shoulders had bent, her tummy had distended, her mouth had tightened and the spring in the dark curls of her hair had become lank. Not only had the colour gone with age, it had gone with the passing of her true being. So I began to describe the nature of my mother as she had been when she was well. I found myself phrasing it, writing it in my mind. I came to the idea; I would write a eulogy to be read at the church service which would paint a picture of the mother I had loved so deeply. I would write with as much skill, compassion, and true love as my talent could muster. After this I slept.

The next day I felt as though I were in shock. Grief was with me; I cried from time to time. I concentrated on my writing. Ben and I found the source of some words that I'd heard in a cathedral in England; Corinthians, Chapter 15, which I had thought were just for me and which talked about the spirit, the passing from one state of being to another. I had heard the words as preparation for myself. Here I was wanting to use them as comfort for those who felt that they had lost my mother. Ben found a small piece from *The Prophet* which talked about grief. I flanked the picture of my mother with that item and the soothing words of St Paul.

As we flew to Mount Gambier I thought of how, if my mother had lived, she would have been coming in the opposite direction to stay with us for a week. I had planned the week so that she and I could do some of the things which she normally couldn't do. I felt stronger too and more able to take her out. But that was not to be. I dreaded seeing Father. At the airport everybody seemed numb. Father clung to me without crying. He was lost and quiet, he wasn't quite here.

That night I heard the train of events from Father, the first of many recountings. It was good to hear Father communicating facts and feelings, like so many symptoms to be expressed. He'd been away that week and had returned on Wednesday to find my mother at the end of a drinking bout, very weak and not well, but she'd insisted that he go again. He'd stayed as late as he could then left her with a cup of tea and several bottles of lemonade. When he came home on Friday night, he couldn't find her. He knew something was wrong. The cup of tea, half drunk, sat on her bedside table.

He ran from room to room turning on lights and calling out, but she was nowhere to be seen. Once more he went to the bedroom and as he tried to push the door back, it resisted. There he found her, crumpled up in her underclothes, one side of her face terribly stained where all the blood had collected and where she'd given herself a terrible knock as she had fallen. He went down on his knees and tried to revive her. In a panic he went to the phone and rang for an ambulance, but half way through the dialling he stopped. "I must be mistaken," he said, "I must be mistaken," talking to himself all the time. He went back and felt her shoulder. "She was stone cold," he said. He put a blanket over her and returned to phone the ambulance. He also rang the mates he'd just left. They came to be with him to wait for the ambulance and the police.

We went to the church service, not knowing if my mother's body had been dissected or had simply been dismissed on the basis of her previous medical history. The details are too confusing and too silly for me to talk about. I was pleased when we drew up to the church twenty minutes early, to see that the coffin was there. We discovered later that my mother's body had been left intact. This was the fourth day by my calculations.

Earlier that morning, Ben and I had talked with Kate about the possibility of her going to the service. Ben explained that some people might be very upset. I added that the ceremony was a way of saying goodbye to Nan. Katie, sitting there with her hands together, feeling this was an important decision and expressing it in the way she spoke said "Well Mummy, crying is a way of saying goodbye, isn't it?" I almost wept. Where did this child come from? Katie came to the ceremony.

We met Dave, a family friend. He was just the right person to read the eulogy I had written, and given to him the previous day. Dave spoke with the strength and the assistance that I knew was with me. His voice was vibrant and sure and he read my words with exactly the right tone and meaning. As I walked out of the church, I felt good in the knowledge that the memory of my mother was restored.

The bursts of grief which I was to know for months after, and even now, were not there with me that day. All day I had beside me the strength of conviction of my mother's rest and peace, and the fact of her still being. I thought of how she was now with my father, my grandparents, Uncle Gordon, little Gavin and all the other loved people who'd been watching over her. That knowledge meant the tears still to be shed weren't close at hand during that day. It was as if a picture of grief was elsewhere, but that the strong picture of my mother being in heaven, as it were, was before my eyes.

When I returned home I found small mementos which reminded me of the week which I would have had with my mother. Mending was on my chair in the bedroom. A letter to be read, a book to be delved into, awaited her. Each one had to be put away. Lying in my bed at night I could almost hear her coming down the hall, speaking in a loud voice, for her hearing had dropped. Speaking right over the top of all of us in her efforts to communicate. I could hear her strong walk in the house, I could smell the warm breath against my cheek, the touch of her hand on my arm, the tremor in those fingers. Her hands had had such character; they were graceful hands, skilful hands, hands which had shown love in the work she did for others, but hands which had lost the art of lovingly touching; the well of love within my mother had begun to dry up from the very day my father died. Now the two of them were dead.

The love which I had learnt to express for my stepfather came through strongly. I rang him often and kept in touch. The bonds that had always been there grew in a way which had never happened before. Father and I supported each other with the picture of my dead mother between us. That picture would fade but it was a link that would always be there. It was a link which joined the life I'd had as a small child with my own blood father, to the life that I later led, at first so unwillingly, with the father who came to us through the choice of my mother.

A dream: The mandala

I stood in a room surrounded by my grandmother's possessions. They were positively riches, treasures to me, they were about to be auctioned and already I felt their loss. Why should others have the right to my grandmother's things simply because they had the money to pay for them? Couldn't I just have two pieces? I decided I would plead my case.

My eye ran round the room listing, evaluating and deciding what meant most to me. As I walked towards a small dais, I decided at least I would have the tapestry firescreen as my grandmother had probably embroidered it herself. That, I thought, would serve a useful purpose for in our new house we had an open fire. I mounted the steps, ran my fingers in a caressing movement over the moulded wood of the balustrade and when I reached the top of the half dozen steps I turned right and found there a lectern. On top, lying in pride of place, was an enormous family Bible which was bound with delicately tooled leather and fine gold leafed embellishments. On the cover was a large symbol, circular with concentric shapes within it and right in the centre it seemed as though it became the pupil of an eye. It also looked as though it contained the letter "I". This book I must also have. This symbol, what does it represent? A mandala — a series of concentric designs representing aspects of one's life, the search for self and one's relationship with the cosmos. The family Bible — testament of goodness, truth and love was the base, the foundation

of my life which my grandmother had given to me. The
cover, the search for self, was my own affair. As I went
down the steps again I decided that the Bible I could
have by right. It was my inheritance. But the safeguard,
the fire screen, was something that I would have to pay
for and bid for myself.

I mused as I woke that this dream should have
been vague and mysterious, yet it was bright and
detailed as though it was an illuminated page of
history come to life in my dream.

20. Sylvia comes to rest. October 1980

I'd never really thought about reincarnation until I
had had that experience of my own past life in
Peter's study. When the idea was first posed, I
neither believed nor disbelieved — it was simply an
interesting thought. I respected those who firmly
held the view of continuing lives, for who was I to
scoff? I was firmly convinced of the after-life, of the
reality of the after-life, so why should I dispute the
idea of a "before-life"? A lecturer in the education of
disturbed children impressed me with his statement
that, although all his experience with those children
pointed in that direction, and although he was a
follower of empirical evidence, his twentieth-century
intellect refused to accept its existence. That's
exactly how I reacted for some time too.

I overheard Katie telling Gollywog when she was

about three, "Poor Grandma, she's very sad because her friend Mr Simons has just died. He's decided to go back to heaven so that he can start to be a baby again."

My little nephew is not much older and his words seem to say the same thing. "Where did you and Daddy live before I came back?", and "Did I come back before you were married or after?"

Katie is now seven. When I showed her my doll, Sylvia, and told her that my Daddy gave it to me for my second birthday, she remarked with perfect calmness that she never knew my Dad and that he had died before she was ready. You may well ask "Ready for what?"

I've been thinking of my dead parents a lot lately. About a month ago Cheryl told me she had rescued Sylvia from going to the rubbish heap when my stepfather was sorting the belongings that he and my mother had shared during their lives together. When she told me that Sylvia only had one arm and was looking very dilapidated, I didn't care — she was still my doll no matter how old and dishevelled.

When I passed on this vital piece of good news to one of my oldest friends I astonished myself by bursting into uncontrollable tears. As I spoke I saw a toddler running from the scene of her mother's violent death, dragging her rag doll behind her; yanking its arm out of its socket. I wandered around all day, dazed and unsettled, trying to understand my streaming grief. The next day I was going to visit Father for a few days to see him settled in his new home with the woman whom I suspected was eventually going to be his new mate. I seemed to have no central reference point . . . even my feet seemed light and groundless. Surely a grown woman who had a perfectly happy marriage, a family and home of her own, shouldn't feel as I was feeling. I described how I felt to my friend on the 'phone again later that day. Hearing the symbolism of my words as I spoke I realized that I was feeling exactly as my mother would feel — alone, replaced, without a home. Once before, when my mother remarried, I had known what it was to have a parent replaced. The tears I had still not shed for my mother's death joined the grief I carried for my own father; the years of not having him by my side, of not knowing what he truly was, my being denied the support of his family background and the cultural inheritance he would have given me. Although the circumstance had been different in my past life, I had experienced exactly the same emotional climate. There my mother had been parted from me, not in death, but in physical distance, and that father had not recognized me as his own. Now it came to me so that the souls of my father and my mother seemed to join with my own in one terrible point of pain.

In an effort to give it salve, Carolyn took me to a wildlife sanctuary nearby, where I could feel the spiritual help that I knew would come to me there. The springs of water which trickled out of the hillside cooled the heat of my emotion and carried the pain from my consciousness. Carolyn had experienced death as hardly anyone is asked to. She had lost brother, uncle, grandmother, cousin, father, and husband in six annual and consecutive deaths. She had told me when my mother died, that the grief never lessened in its intensity, but that the periods between its expression grow longer.

The sense of being which the glistening rocks and water gave to me seemed to take me into the timeless aspects of the earth — to give back to me the perspective of my transient life.

I went off the next day to give my approval to the changes that Father was making. All went well except for a brief spell when my nephew plunged me into his feelings and my own again. Cheryl, too, was finding it difficult and didn't seem to be able to bring the meaning of death to her young son. On the first visit to Nan's grave to place some flowers, Andrew had hurried to the gardener's shed, saying "Here Mummy — Nan's waiting in there for me. Hurry up, she'll be glad to see me . . . she hasn't seen me for a long time."

Cheryl retold this episode to me as we approached the grave and again when Father was snipping the grass from around the memorial plaque and shining it up with baby oil, Andrew asked "What's the matter Pa? Can't you find her?" All the longing to understand the meaning of death, which had haunted my child's heart came back to me as sharp as a stabbing knife.

On the way home in the train, away from Father's new beginnings, I prayed for rest, my ears almost deaf to Katie's happy chatter. At last the links were made and peace returned. As I nursed my seven-year-old to sleep in my arms, I relished the form of her warm, live body, rhythmically moving against me in sleep. So far she at least was safe in the expressed love of two live parents and the doting attentions of several surviving grandparents.

Just before bed the next evening, Katie caught sight of Sylvia lying on my bedroom cupboard, naked and unattended. I don't know how, but Sylvia's arm is now intact; her wig is gone but the neat moulded shape of her hair is there. At one stage as a child, I washed away her painted face, and years later her china features show through with simple clarity. The sockets of her eyes are blank; her blue eyes, disconnected, lie inside her head, looking inwards.

"I won't take her away for long" said Katie, "I know she's too precious."

Back Sylvia came, her thin grubby body dressed in a little flowered frock, socks on her rag legs cut out of Katie's brand new tights, her bare head nestling in a little hand-made bonnet which Aunty Vera had knitted for me as a baby and which had graced her babies' heads as well. "I'll just make her a bed" said Kate. Sylvia was wrapped in a crocheted rug and put to sleep back on the cupboard, her head resting on a pillow Kate had made for her own doll. Katie did not know that she had laid Sylvia on a wrapped photograph that Father had given me. The photograph was my parents on their wedding day.

"Mummy" said Kate "she's got a very dirty face, and she hasn't got any eyes, but you know she's really quite beautiful."

I slept well. Kate didn't notice that Sylvia's crying mechanism was broken and nor did she know that the faces of my dead parents did not appear in my dreams that night. They still looked towards each other on the cupboard, smiling with happiness, stepping out of the church door into the sunlight. Together again, I thought. We drifted into our various states of rest. I lost the vision of the arum lilies that lay in my mother's arms.

A dream: Hiding the child away

*"I don't think the mother should have left this child
with me — she should have taken it with her."*

*"I wonder if I can pick her up? I can't bear to hear
a child crying."*

"I will. I am going to pick her up."

*It took some time to find the frail little crumpled body
lying in foetal position in the dust. Everything here was
gloomy and ill-defined, hard to bring into focus. As I
picked up the child her limbs fell downwards like the
limp legs and arms of a rag doll. There seemed little life
and little form remaining in her body. As I encircled
her in my arms pressing her close, it seemed she was
almost as cold as clay. If only my body warmth could
surge into her, that my own warm streaming blood could
be transfused into her own. If only I could fill the limp
and flaccid body with warm mother's milk. If only my
eyes could seek the gaze that now was turned inwards
behind the closed lids. I instinctively cradled her back
against my warm stomach and pulled her head towards
my breast. But my breast was gone and the breast that
remains is dry. I cannot give her all that she needs.
Who can I ask for this food?*

21. The battle continues

Before me is a book with pictures of warriors. They are men of war of ancient times. They have very warm brown skin, not black but rather like the Polynesians. The setting is not the jungle or the tropics — it is more like an uncultivated English countryside. The men are dressed in skins, bare-armed and bare-legged, and decorated with many signs of initiation: long welts, scars line their chests and their hair is drawn back in a ritual band.

As I watch, a giant of a man starts towards me. I don't know what kind of warrior he is?" asks someone who is reading the manual with me. "I don't know and I don't have time to work it out, but he looks a little like a Maori." I almost panic as he continues to rise up out of the book towards me. Suddenly I am backed against a high barricaded fence, but although I know that safety and peace lie on the other side, it is not right for me to escape. As I stand against this high wall of finely tied trees, I don't have time to arm myself or to defend myself. The warrior cuts off my legs with one mighty sweep of his scythe-like sword.

That's how I feel about the cancer at this stage. I seem today almost as though I can hardly keep in balance. Somehow I felt that if I could not defeat it, at least I could keep it at bay. Now, here I am, with a lump in my breast, another lump, which is as active as a hundred little knife-bearing people inside the spot in my flesh, and it feels as though they are all wearing their blades on small dancing feet. Three angry red spots have appeared in the centre of my left breast, one bigger than the rest. At first I felt they were merely something that the homoeopathics were bringing to the surface, to be expressed. But still they get larger, more defined and harder in the centre. I have to be thankful for the fact that my organs are free, but the four small spots of cell activity on my bones worry me and have sapped my confidence. It seems like an all-round attack on my being: an attack on my thinking with the two spots in my temples; the spots in the discs in the centre of my spine will affect my uprightness; in my hips, my mobility; and in my ribs, my breathing. It was no news that something was wrong. It seems we were given a week to prepare ourselves while we waited for the results of the scan. While the X-ray plates, inaccessible to us, were locked away in some uncaring secretarial closet while the doctor took an inconvenient holiday, Ben and I tried to brace ourselves to face a new situation. Up to this stage the hope of getting completely well was still quite realistic.

When eventually the doctor carefully went through each plate, Ben and I sat in what must have been shock. Throughout the week we had been passively waiting — now our hearts beat fast, our hands were moist within each other's clasp. "Why couldn't he have read them first and broken the news to me cleanly and quickly?" It reminded me of how I had been in Peter's room when I had followed the imagery of the warriors and how in that much earlier time I had discovered, and indeed experienced, death. In the image I had been a warrior still strong, like the Maori who had killed me in the dream. As a warrior I had been mutilated and captured in battle. My spirit had escaped, but my body had lived on, despite its cruel cuts and the humiliation of the treatment I experienced at the hands of my captors. They were eager to see how much a great hulk of a body could endure, and how much it would take to kill finally the body itself. In that life, that experience, that consciousness (call it what you like — maybe it's all three together) the only escape I could find was into insanity.

In my last life I had escaped into death and found the healing of the angels. Now it seems there is no escape from conscious pain. Here I am with so much that I want to achieve but with a body this time which is letting me down: which is expressing the effects of war, the feelings of attack I had as a child, not just on behalf of my father but also for myself — expressing the war in an inner way and then out through my body which is manifesting the cancer. There is a key, somewhere, to the healthy expression of all the previous pain and hurt. If only I could find it, the hurts could fly free from my body like birds from a cage. I thought that I was doing everything that could lead me to health again, but now I feel that the ground has been cut away from beneath me.

One night during my meditation, an old man came round the edge of the bed to stand at my side. I hardly dare speak of such things, but this man offered his help. He appeared to me not as a bright vision in a dream, nor as a dark but visible shape in the room. His form was filled with a faintly glowing and moving light but I could see the physical outlines of my bedroom behind his shape. It was as if I could see life without a physical body. I found myself thinking "My God. This is what people have described, or have imagined as ghosts." Somehow, even though he fitted what has become a trivial image viewed with scorn and scepticism, he was real enough for me to be filled with awe and overcome with feelings of inadequacy. I had heard of spiritual guides before and I neither accepted nor discounted the phenomenon. I have had enough experience of the kind that cannot be substantiated, which is neither the acceptance of the belief nor the acquiring of factual knowledge, to feel quite open to any idea if it becomes a demonstrated reality. Nevertheless like a stupid, insecure child I sent him away saying that at this stage I did not know what it was that I needed to know — and now I cannot find him.

It was my sense of not being worthy of such special treatment that made me turn him away.

I lost an opportunity to gain knowledge in a direct way. It is as though on one hand we can deal directly with our wise and constructive selves, or else choose to bring consciousness and therefore wisdom through actual physical states or experiences of the body. There is real experience, not just thoughts and ideas, between me and the realization of what healing entails. Perhaps there is a need to die first. I hardly know where these thoughts come from, I hardly know if I should be penetrating my understanding of this life more fully, so as to keep a grasp on what is happening to me, or whether instead I should be loosening the threads very gradually so that death can come more easily to me this time. I am no longer trying to fight someone, but instead there is support to give me rest, to give me succour, while I lick my new wounds.

Along with the warming food, I have been given some warming medicine, and I have begun taking rosemary baths, and best of all, Ben is learning to give me massage. His large hands can give me an etheric wall to keep in the warmth I'm managing to manufacture.

Meanwhile I'm sure the Iscador will gather itself again now that it is being supported. For my routine, with my music, with my eurythmy, all those creative forces which have been going haywire, pleasing themselves in fact, must be affected and harmonized to some extent.

In the past I felt as if I was fighting alone, or almost alone. Except for the considerable help that Dr Twentyman gave me it seemed I had to organize my own healing, my own medicine. The rift between what was acceptable to me and the aggressive orthodox methods for treating cancer was so great, there seemed to be little I could do besides the Iscador and the general homoeopathy which was directly related to my individual needs.

It seems strange that one of the prospective users of Iscador whom I visited should find for me a doctor who is willing to draw the two streams of medicine together. How good it feels for someone with present-day knowledge and an open mind to present to me options for my new position. So here I am trying a new drug, which ironically Dr Twentyman suggested two years ago. It was not available here at the time.

I feel that I am gathering my own strength, but with the support of other forces at last. I no longer have to fight it almost single-handed. How much of that situation did I orchestrate for myself and how much help is there if we only know how and where to seek it? It seems that every one of us who wishes to take hold of, and be responsible for the direction of their lives must consciously find deep within their own being (or is it outside?) the source of their own life. That source is not related to war, but is exactly the opposite. This search could be likened (if we used an ancient allegory) to the search for the Holy Grail — not seen as a far-flung journeying but a penetration to the unique self, right here in our own frames. Why do I think that we have to make that journey so that every dying child can be sustained?

My initiation continues. How many scars on my breast will complete the test? How much blood needs to warm the battleground at my feet, before our mutual goals are one? Still the arrows let out the blood, still the bullets and the bombs perforate the body and blow it to smithereens and still I cling to my image of the breast transforming blood to life-giving milk. What is the meaning of the image of the warrior with a sword in his hands? If we wield the sword and let out blood, does this lead us any further in our search for the meaning of blood itself? I keep hearing like a pulse in my being, "The blood of Christ, The blood of Christ, The blood of Christ."

22. Winter 1981

Today I've had a revelation. The last time I felt my position was hopeless was the night before I had the first session of general tests and my first radio isotope and scan two and a half years ago. I remember that night ringing Marlene and saying to her that I had no sense of my future, no sense of light or of hope. I almost felt that I was in the state of the living dead. I was deeply shocked at the thought that we had just arranged a new section of our lives, we had at last made arrangements for Katie to go to her most special school, we'd spent two years building a house which would be supportive to the values and life-style we felt that a young child should have and which was right for ourselves as well. And then came the blow of knowing I had another tumour. In the previous months I had worked very hard in what I call my political life, and I felt that in fact I had given away far more of myself than I actually had to give. I felt as though I had been paying a price for something that I couldn't have, atoning for things that I really didn't know about, trying to earn my place in life and, of course, these are barters that just cannot be made. Marlene said to me that I must just have trust, that to trust in the direction of your life no matter what it might be, is something that inevitably everybody must face. We have to give up the idea of being in the driver's seat — like the picture that had so appealed to me in the past, of a rider in charge of her surfboard and making use of the waves to go in the direction that she had chosen for herself. But here I was overwhelmed. I seemed to have no choice, no say; and the direction was obscured. It was at this time too that I had many dreams of avalanching waves coming into my house. Marlene's words of comfort brought more than just the ideas. They brought with them a conviction of the stance that she took, and I trusted her so deeply I was able to face the night knowing that she was supporting me.

Over the past two weeks I have managed to wrap myself in a cloak of anaesthesia, a cloak of my own making. This of course has not prevented me from thinking. I have faced my death. I have faced the possibility of dying within months of this time, and then I received the news that the spread of my cancer is, in fact, still manageable to some degree. Now that means that I can never again regain full strength, but there is the possibility of making my life last a little longer. I've not allowed myself to hope. Before the results I could hardly bear the thought that perhaps I simply had a breast tumor, a fourth breast tumour. I could not trust to such enormous luck. This was a realistic assessment, I know, but it seems sad to relate that I still cannot bear that kind of optimism. Still — even after all the lessons — I invest all the power, all the strength in myself. And because I do this, all the blame lies within me. I've tried desperately to give up the burden, to say, "Here I am, take me as I am, help me to walk beside you instead of taking the lead". If only I could find that trust.

I'm not afraid of dying at all. I know this life is

a preparation for a task that is awaiting me, and I know that I've chosen a very difficult time of learning. The silly thing is, I could have taken on that task in this life, if only I'd had the courage to trust in the right course of events. At least now I know that Ben and Kate will survive without me in a way that will be right for them, but I grieve so terribly for the fact that I'd wanted to make Ben really happy. When we married he told me that he'd not cared about tomorrow and I wanted to contribute to his life in a way that would bring him joy and make him want to live every day as fully as possible. He certainly lived that life, with a consciousness that he didn't have before. But why did that consciousness bring such dreadful pain? I already feel his grief, and sometimes the pain of parting is almost too strong for me to bear. Until yesterday I'd kept these feelings quite at bay. I had been living on a level slightly above the earth and apart from those I love, but yesterday I came back.

Here I am again. Every minute is excruciatingly painful and joyous at the same time. Kate's little voice singing at the organ, with the ear phones on, as she accompanies herself comes to me like the air that I'm breathing. It fills me up. Her little body sitting on my knee is so real it's overwhelming. There are quieter comforts too, lying in the warmth of a comfortable bed with Ben's strong body beside me, breathing rhythmically in his sleep, offering a hand as he turns in the bed. The strong warmth he exudes is in contrast to the struggling of my body just to keep its own temperature. The cold of the night comes in through the window and invades.

I have no armour. I am at the mercy of all that

comes to me and so Ben's warmth is like a lifeline; I live in the aura of his existence at this time.

As I meditate on the words "God has given the sun for the healing of mankind. The great sun of the Godhead reposes within us, its rays penetrate to heaven from where they came," I see this as a living picture.

It is true, I am sure, that cancer is a non-working of the warmth mechanism in our being — and that means through our whole being — not just physical warmth. If I can make myself open to that mechanism being restored, repaired, brought back into harmony, I can be healed. But to have that ray of hope, that stream of living golden light to offer myself to, requires a strength, a concentration of consciousness that I know is almost beyond my ability at this stage. I will try but I know now that I can't manufacture that feeling for myself. It is not something that I can produce, it is something I must aid and help make myself open to.

The paradox of the situation is that it is only with the consciousness which comes with the experience that my cancer has brought, that I can understand and know the nature of healing. So I must simply be satisfied with the thought that that knowledge is worthwhile in itself, even though I may not bear the fruit of that knowledge. At least I will carry that with me for my next life, and it can be used productively in the way in which I tackle the task that I know is waiting for me.

All these thoughts sustain me. But I know the feelings must be met and must be dealt with. The harmony that I must reach again must be worked for. So you see there is work to be done but not all the work is mine. That brings me both a sense of ease and a sense of 'dis-ease'.

I cannot simply remain divorced, apart, in the realm of thought. I have to meet death in life with all of my being, it must be consciously, fully, trustingly and faithfully experienced. I suppose I am being offered the ultimate agony and ecstasy of which I have so often thought. Now I can understand how the act of thought brings things into being.

I will now meditate on the power of warmth, of love, of light, of sun, and of life and my relationship to it.

23. Isis

I S I S. These letters shimmer in ice-blue light in the normally blank space behind my closed eyelids. I was meditating, asking for guidance. I seemed to be stumped, in some kind of impasse in my search for understanding of my disease. All the working through in this life (the so called "shocking experience" in my past life which had ended in my death — violent and sudden), seemed to have been achieved. I could understand; the loss of breath in the asthma, and the choking feelings that came with it. Then there was the loss of my sight, the slashing of eyes and breast, the feelings of panic that came out in this life as tachycardia. But these bones — in that life I had no broken bones. What did it mean?

"What do you know about Isis," Peter asked me in the next therapy.

"Well, all I know is that she was an Egyptian goddess of some kind. Actually, the blue of the writing was the same kind of blue you associate with their temple frescoes . . . perhaps she's a goddess of love?"

"Do you know anything else?"

"No," I replied, thinking hard.

Silence.

"Well, what comes to mind about the letters themselves?"

"When I first saw it, it seemed to be almost two words. IS IS. Like two states of being — the physical life and the spiritual life. And then of course the "I" seems to be for the self, upright and individual."

"And the 'S'?"

"Oh . . . somehow it seems to have both the aspect of the snake and also a sense of fitting together: the top and the bottom are like a mirror image, or two sides of the question, or even the same question put another way."

"What does the snake bring to mind?"

"It reminds me of the snake in the Garden of Eden, of course; the loss of innocence, like the loss of innocence I experienced when I discovered that this world would kill a little child's father. And with the coming of knowledge, there is the thought that we must then stop being children and take our own future in our hands."

Another thinking quietness came as Peter and I digested all of this.

At last Peter asked, "Have you never heard of the legend of Isis and Osiris?"

"I've never heard of Osiris," I said.

He told me that Isis and Osiris were husband and wife, deeply devoted to each other. Osiris had a brother who was as evil as Osiris was good. He was envious of Osiris and so he slew him. Isis had the power to bring the dead to life with her love and so this she did with her lover. Osiris's brother slew Osiris again and in a rage he cut the body into a million pieces and flung them the length of the Nile. Poor Isis spent the remainder of her life searching for the pieces. All were found but the phallus — the symbol of fertility and continuing adult life."

I was stunned. How I could still marvel at the things that Peter and I unearthed together I can't imagine, but I did.

. . . the cancer had taken my fertility; and the inability to find my father as a true personality, my inability somehow to realize the relationship of daughter and father, had taken my freedom to relate to normal, adult love that is sexual. The cancer had also taken from me the spontaneous nature of my rich physical love which I had experienced with Ben. Now, I had almost to dig myself out of a straight-jacket to break open the cache of response that I knew was there.

This revelation had other meanings too.

A short time later, in a reverie which was in quality a meditation unsought, I found myself thinking again of the circumstances of my father's death. In my mind, I saw the jeep drive along the narrow, tortuous road in the New Guinea mountains. I then saw the jeep blow up. A million pieces of debris rained in the air. I saw it like a slow motion film, without sound. There was a sound inside me nevertheless — the deep, pushing action of my heart, pushed a tide of blood into my ears.

Here I was alive, watching in retrospection, my father's untimely exploding into another state. The unfilled picture of my childhood, where there had been no action — just a sudden stop and then blank until now when I pictured my father's body lying in a coffin. I had been told that he had died instantly, and I had heard them talking.

"They drove into a land mine . . . Nothing recognizable left, but the steering wheel."

And the truth came to me in stark, unmistakable clarity — my father would have been blown to pieces in that act of war. As a little child I was not silly. Could I have ingested that horrible, deeply shocking reality . . . have unconsciously worked it out . . . and unable to bear it, locked it away? I know that reality cannot be locked away or rubbed out of our eternal picturing. There it must have been all these years . . . a moving, live picture in my soul — demanding response, emitting signals like a hidden guerilla post . . . affecting my life and poisoning it with dreadful feelings too large until now to let flow.

My bones, I thought. Those feelings were right deep into my bones. And then I could see my own body, like my father's, being shattered, broken apart. All these spots in my bones, in my skeleton, are like an image of my father's. If only I could find those feelings again. It's like an operation to be performed. Could it be done, for the parts affected were my own framework?

. . . Thinking more about it I felt that as a small child, your life's patterning, your life's energy, is so tied to your parents, that if their direction, or image is broken, so is your own. Perhaps the damage that was done to my father's body, was registered somehow on my own.

Later I put aside everything to meditate in a special way for my father. I knew that his spiritual being would now be intact, but at the time of the explosion his physical body would have so suddenly disintegrated that it must have seemed that his spirit was expelled like a puff of smoke. It was as though my father had become so insubstantial in my memory and my imagination, that he had simply been blown away — like ashes from a blazing inferno. I must, like Isis, try to find him. First in meditation I would find his form. I knew about the healing that comes after death, when spiritual beings bring to form, bring back again, the perfect healthy body that is essentially yours. Now, in my imagination I gathered the pieces of my father's body from the surrounds of the accident, and with loving hands, placed them in his coffin. I saw it seal together and then, while as a whole body, it slowly became dust, in that world where there is no time, no space, . . . where there is light that heals, and all is love, . . . I saw my father's form intact. My fingers joined the fingers of the spiritual form bringing him back to himself. Of course, as I have said, this had already been done I am sure, but I had to take part in it so that it became real to me also.

Auntie Vera heard I was not well and came to stay. Her stay was so important. We laughed and talked for hours. She insisted that I spend every minute she was here doing exactly what I wanted. She was a great impetus for my writing. She gave me the time and also she brought to mind some forgotten scenes from childhood and in those scenes she portrayed my father, large as life. He was the bright urbane young man I had imagined — generous and full of promise. I found it hard to realize that unlike me, he was a night bird who loved to sleep in after working half the night. After Auntie Vera had helped at my birth, my mother had sent her in to wake up my father so that he could look at his first child.

"Six o'clock!" he said. "What an ungodly hour to greet a child for the first time!" He rolled over to catch up on his sleep. Did he love me as I loved him? Surely you don't experience a love so great if it is unnurtured by its recipient.

. . . Time after time I have imagined I have eventually laid my father to rest, but again and again another piece of the puzzle turns up. I may have picked up the pieces of his broken body, but still it seems the puzzle is not yet solved. Until it is I cannot get better and perhaps I cannot manage that in this lifetime.

24. The passing of dark blood

The night wore a hood of unleavened cloud. A desultory breeze scattered dead leaves about the feet of scarcely moving trees. Inside, in bed, the woman lay tense, her nerves singing and taut as electric wires strung from poles in the countryside.

She felt like screaming and as she felt it within her, she screamed inside. She screamed loud and long with as much force as an inside scream will allow.

"Why am I screaming?" her small inside voice asked.

Then into the screaming came the feeling, the feeling of absolute, overwhelming terror. Inside herself she tried to break free of it, but she could not, and with that realization came the feeling of being overcome. She was being overcome, she was trapped, and into the experience she disappeared: A man was struggling to hold her still, wishing to overpower her to devour her in some way. She screamed and screamed for help. Desperately she screamed for her lover to come, for he might be a match for this brute. He did not come, she was abandoned. His strength was more than physical and here she was fighting for her life with unequal power. Why should she be asked to fight for her life with abilities she did not possess? She was not only at a disadvantage, she was lost.

For an instant the sight of the knife, a flashing dagger, caught her eye and for that instant she contemplated grabbing it from her assailant through some cunning

trick, but with that brief contemplation came the realiz-
ation that she would have to kill to save her own life.
She would have to kill, or be killed. She could not do
it. This was an unfair fight. Not all the self-knowledge,
not all the painful journey and transforming of a
hundred lives, not all her capacity to love and seeking
of the good. . . . not any of her strivings could come to
her aid. There had been no preparation for killing, only
that knife grasped in her hands and struck deep into the
heart of her assailant could save her.

She gave up to inevitable death. She lay in her
captor's arms, unconscious, limp, impotent and already
beyond his reach.

Always before when I have described this experience
to Peter or to myself, I had relived it a little, like a
sleep walker. I had felt myself slipping into unconsciousness, I had felt a terrible racking grief for my
departure and my leave-taking of the lover and child
of those times. I had almost moaned at the unbidden
interruption of a happy life. That life had the quality
of spring flowers, the consistency of creamy butter,
but it had ended with the stains of darkening blood
on the floor of the deserted cellar.

I felt emptied of disquieting emotion, released
again, I fell at last into restorative sleep knowing
that I would not wake waiting to hear the stealing
footsteps that had followed me in another life.

A possum jumped on to the iron roof, a bird
stirred in the leaves and gave a small sound of dis-
turbance. The clouds moved on, thinning until only
a soft mist hid the outlines of the sharp white moon.

The next afternoon the scar on my left breast was
sharp and deep with pain. It took some time to draw

it together enough for me to begin my meditation. It had been paining all day in a dull, cotton-wool kind of way, but now it had flared to a rich, red flame. As my concentration centred on the pain, it seemed to draw together in a cloud, and as I spoke my mantram rhythmically with the beat of my heart, the pain changed to a warm, almost hot cloud which hovered above my breast and its river like a scar. Then, as I watched with my meditating sense, it rose like a moving flood of blood, richly red, up through my throat, enveloping my head until it passed straight up and away from me. This flowing, easy passage from me had clouded my vision, as if washed through my eyes. A moment's disquiet gave way to a bemused interest. I felt that I had been a spectator in some strange procedure. Again I felt a sensation of relief and release.

My meditation went on. It became more like a quiet contemplation which ended in sleep.

25. The fire opens my eyes

It was summer, a few years ago. Kate and I, bare-limbed in the warmth, were walking to a neighbour's house in a nearby street. Every now and then a gum tree would mark its presence by its tang of eucalyptus hanging in the air. Kate was up ahead of me, travelling twice my distance as she skipped and danced from discovery to discovery. By the time we reached our destination, I knew her pockets and mine would be full of her "finds" — small evidences of how beautiful she found the world.

"Mum," she said coming back towards me, "do you remember how blue the sky can be?"

"Oh yes," I said, immediately up there in my mind.

"Well," she said, skirting my moving cane to take my hand, "you know the kind of blue it would be on a lovely summer day? Well, it's like that and its all decorated with little white clouds."

"I know," I said.

Above me the blue became a mantle billowing high and wide, its colour like unending love. This was a perfect day . . . a day that was a gift of nature and Kate in her painting of it for me in her words, was as clear as she could have been with her paint brush and paper.

During the same summer (she must have been six) she and I were on the deck, enjoying the sun again. As I lay, lost in my thoughts, Kate chattered and pottered about, watering the flowers and shifting things to her own order. Then there was an intense silence. I waited, then quietly asked, "What are you doing?"

Slowly came the answer.

"I'm just looking at this butterfly. You know Mum," she said in her "educating Mum" voice, "anyone would think this was just an ordinary orange and black butterfly, but it's not! If you really look you can see that it's not just plain black — it's a bluish black, a brownish black, a yellowish black, and a greyish black . . . you know, actually" (she emphasised *actually* as though introducing a long lost friend) "this butterfly has a beautiful design."

"Design" I thought. That's such a precise word for a young child to use. My imagination let loose. "*De*-sign," I thought, "sign off" . . . what? "*Deo*-sign" flashed before me, "sign of God"!

It seemed to me that children and nature were the source of much understanding and knowledge. Kate was actually leading me to look beyond the ordinary or trivial appearance of things to penetrate the meaning. This winter as I sat before the fire trying to write a poem for her, trying to catch the essential nature of winter, I found myself looking at everything as merely a covering . . . a sheath to be penetrated.

As I sat before the fire working in this way, I saw the symbol of the phoenix . . . the transformed form from the burning, rising up as spirit towards heaven.

I wonder if the dead are watching. I wonder if in these times when the outer work of the earth is so still, they feel in closer contact with us.

The ticking of the old clock continued from the mantel-shelf as the flames of the fire died down. I wonder who will be waiting for me when I die? Almost an army of faces appeared before me — my father, my mother, all my grandparents, Uncle Gordon with his son Gavin, my adolescent friend Judy, Kit, and Shirley who was the first of the long train of those who have died of cancer. This group of cancer casualties, I may have met only once or twice but when you are dying together, your words and contact are straight and deep.

I thought of my own spiritual body and felt that in these activities I was making the fabric of it stronger, denser in my innermost place of being. I could see it like a column of white light within me, a column of uprightness that acted like a plumb bob to all my movements.

Soon it will be spring, I thought. I will take the ashes of the fire then, and place them on the rose bed. It will be feed for the new flowering. The fire, the phoenix, the ashes and the flowers. My eyes had travelled a long way this night. I had begun with the seemingly empty winter landscape and here I was contemplating another flower, another spring. We are lucky, I thought, here in the southern hemisphere — we have spring and the Easter imagination flanking the length of the winter.

Meantime the winter wind is bracing. — Actually, as Kate would say, 'bracing is exactly the right word'. At teachers' college our insignia was the rising phoenix, and its motto, *"Through strength to the stars"*. The winter and the work it leads us to do, is not just a separation for our death, for the loss of our physical life, for as our physical body falls away, we brace ourselves and make preparation for existence beyond death.

"Per ardua ad astra"

Auntie Vera rang this morning. I told her that my bones were showing the progression of the cancer. Her usually light happy voice became retracted somehow, as she hid behind it in pain. How I wish I could save my loved ones some of the pain. At one time I thought we were inevitably alone but now I see that we inevitably share each other's joys and difficulties.

As I spoke to Peter of my father, I saw him warm and alive, his face mobile and full of personality, his head upright and bright, topped with his dark auburn hair. But when I looked closer, he became my father in a photograph I have of him; his pose static, his head bent towards my mother, with a hand poised on her shoulder. I tried to catch his attention. He looked up, then with severe gravity he put his hand out to me. I felt my hand enclosed in his and instantly I became a tiny child of indiscernible age. I nestled into his head and shoulder — there I was again, loved, safe, quiet, with my mother and my father. It seemed the right place for me. Into those secure warm feelings came a warning of what happened next . . . the separation, the loss, then grief inexpressible. I could not bear to look a moment more. Peter and I talked about it but it had come too soon after a heavy day.

"Here we see again," he said, "another instance of you becoming so involved in your earthly work that you spend valuable strength for that when it should be used for your inner growth. Perhaps you are really running away from your own inner needs."

I felt more that I was working myself into life. And the beckoning of my dead father was to the child I put aside, and that I must experience in all its devastating agony, the inner being I locked away in a cave out of harm's way — out of life . . . an image reminding me of a mother sheep standing astride her new-born lamb, bleating against calls of the slowly circling crows.

Perhaps, in wanting so desperately to live (in my conscious mind anyway) I am uselessly railing against my destiny. Perhaps my father is truly beckoning me to the spiritual world because it is time.

Perhaps I have learned all I need or can in this life, and it is time for that essential Maxene who lived most fully and truly in the years before the war, to re-emerge in death. Did I, as Marlene suggests, deny my destiny early, in an effort to live more deeply, more consciously into the things that would train me for that same role in another life? Am I one of hordes of people specially preparing through their illness for a more conscious age? It all sounds too much. All that I know is that I don't know. All I feel is impending loss. There are no nurses to hurry up, no antidote to take, and all my strivings will not bring me life. Just now, on a perfect spring day, I am not consoled by the thought of a special pre-paration for a spiritual life. The spiritual world is very real to me, but I want to help to bring it more to earth. I want to get better, I want a new life on earth. The air I breathed seemed full with grace and yet as I sit here with spring entering every part of me, I must prepare for death. Could it be that I haven't found a way to say good-bye to the dead? But that is work; I am tired again and it seems not to be of use. There is only grace, and that I cannot plead or earn — if something isn't freely given, it is not a gift.

A contemplation: My father beckons.

My father beckons . . . My dead father stands before me with hand outstretched, "Stay your hand for I will not come and join you yet." My heart is sore, my body feels hurt, bruised, torn and the space inside me feels raw.

What has been an idealized relationship with a dead parent . . . has it been a forty-year commitment to a father who played being "Daddy" with all the sincere wish to do what he thought was right . . . but who saw me only as a "dear little thing, a doll, a toy . . . not a cherished 'me'." I was separate, with my own future, my own feelings, I was not a reflection of that "going places young man." I was distinctively me . . . not an amalgam of Max and Zena, not Maxene, but me . . . But where is my name? . . . Can I keep that name?

I withdrew, walking backwards from his hand, on my sturdy, if thin legs . . . and as I move back towards my present, his warm face, his auburn hair, his flesh loses shape and colour. There is death before my eyes . . . There is nothing left but bones . . . shining bones, glistening white and whole.

Can my bones restore themselves to a white and glistening state, not ready to dry and disintegrate but flowing with warm blood, its marrow manufacturing its daily army of white knights, waiting to swarm in my blood through the whole of my body —

This army is my army, wearing my insignia, as the white cells carry our finger prints, my army is me — my own salvation, my own resuscitation is in my very bones, stronger than the cancer that is now scattered like pieces of discarded shrapnel.

What is the insignia? Is it Maxene? Has that name become mine despite the names that inhabit it . . . ?

26. The beginning of the end

Each scan has limited my idea of how much life I have left. Has it now changed from an expected couple of years to only a matter of months? How can I say "only a matter of months"? That's my precious life I'm talking about — that's the time I've got left with Ben and my little Kate, with friends and all those people I love. Loving isn't something that belongs to the past. It is always a predictable part of the future. Word travels fast, and yesterday, only hours after I had heard that my spine, my pelvis, my hip, my ribs, my skull were all showing the dark shadows of the blood-consuming cancer, the phone didn't stop ringing, friends arrived, flowers — even the parcels man from Australia Post sent me his love — and out of the blue came a phone call from the woman radiologist who was of course the first to see X-ray pictures of malevolent growth. People come continuously into my life and many remain to share what we have to give to each other.

I was overwhelmed with the love that came flowing to me yesterday. But there is a part of me that almost resents it, while the black picture of cruel circumstance sits in my unconscious. I can feel angry, badly done by, resentful, and in the process I could get rid of the pus that is past bad feelings that have been worked upon, killed off, but not yet expressed through my bodily processes, all that is left to do is the washing and the cleansing of the wound. Yet again I read my words and think it is a description of my illness and proffer the conclusion that I have to die at this stage to heal my "I", my spiritual self. I can't help crying at all the anguish of the disappointment, the let-down, the "I wanted to achieve that in life". Do the gods think me greedy? I wanted so much to finish my book for I know that my life has brought me experience — not just for myself but for many who have travelled with me. Last night my neighbour was comforting me with the vision of an everlasting journey more brilliant and marvellous than we could dream about. I've seen it already in small fragments in my meditations, but last night while Brian was speaking I could only see it, not feel it. At this very moment every ounce of my being is yelling to live. I can't believe that I have to die soon. I couldn't believe it when I was told my eyes would go blind, but gradually, at a rate I could just cope with, they did. The only way I can see again is to die. Is that what I secretly want? My dreams haven't said so. And again my dreams have said I've decided to stay; in another dream I saved the child my mother refused, and in another, all that I had invested in my dead father was given over to Ben. My unconscious has never

189

been more optimistic, still sometimes frightened a little, but never healthier. Isn't it the seat of government? I can still be amazed at what knowledge it can bring me. It is as Jung described: a pathway to the collective knowledge that lives who knows where — Jung thought in the spiritual world. The spiritual is of course the unconscious, the non-physical knowledge that comes in our meditations, our prayers, our dreams.

I wanted to tell Ben how much our life together has been a salve, a rich meal of human experience. As we lie in each other's arms weeping and already dying a little, I feel our love imprinting its existence somewhere. Love actually is the only thing that lasts, a kind of well-spring from where it is expressed into physical form.

All this is so heady. All I want is to lie with my belly, heart and head on soft earth, feeling myself a link between heaven and earth so that I can draw life long enough for me to get used to the idea of dying.

The beautiful drawing that Kate gave me should be all I need. Two streams of flowing water come from both myself and Ben to form her own which drops down in a waterfall, energised and clear into a meadow where the flowers grow in profuse colour, upright and strong. In my part of the river she has given me "a bridge, Mummy, in case you want to cross"; on the other side there is a meadow serene and beautiful.

The night we got the news she remarked: "If Mummy dies she'll be in a safe place, and a safe place is the best place to be."

"All day my eyes kept watering and I couldn't

even remember how to spell" she told Ben, but already a dream she has had tells me that she has a picture of me watching over her when I am dead. In the dream she could see me: well and strong and able to see, wearing a magic ring. Whenever Kate was in trouble I could turn the ring and prevent her being caught or injured. How is it that some children seem to come with wisdom, and already established knowledge?

There is much to be grateful for. I have decided I can't just lie in bed feeling that every day it seems to get worse, so now I will have to achieve one thing out of bed per day. There is nothing more I can do for myself. We all seem to have done all that we can. Now I will simply finish off as many loose ends as I can, write as much of my book as I can, and try to express as much grief for the life I cannot have, in a way that will cause minimal pain to others; if I can do that, I might be able to meet death peacefully or even with some sense of the great journey. Meanwhile, time that has no meaning after death is the all-encompassing ruler of thoughts and feelings. With each day, I have only weeks not months; and then I'll only have days. How cruel that now I can actually see the future again, and now that I have come home to my true self and to so many whom I love and cherish, I should have to give it all up. This is no sacrifice I am making. It is a wrenching, tearing, blood-letting parting over which I no longer have any control.

As I climbed into the hospital bed last week I felt very strongly that I didn't want to die in such a bed. It was narrow and sensible and nothing to do with my life. If only I could die at home. During that week, when I could only sleep for two hours at a time I slipped in and out of meditation and I prayed a great deal. On one occasion I had a sense, just a brief glimpse, of what Christ must feel for others, the love that he must feel. To feel love from that giving viewpoint was almost overwhelming. It was like an explosion of light right in the centre of your being. Now that I've experienced it I can never be the same.

You don't actually die all of a sudden. Not in a situation like mine. I've been loosening threads of my life for years, and especially since last May. Your life gradually dies around you — one part after another is lost, and you realize there are some things that you've already done for the last time.

As I moved further and further into my inner being during my hospital stay, which is quite astounding when you think of the circumstances, I could feel myself consciously letting go of life. That doesn't mean giving it up, but rather letting go that tenacious clawing, "I've got to live at any price". And with that knowledge of slipping into another sphere, or into the spirit, there comes a peace because then time has no meaning; when the beginning and when the end of your life comes is no longer relevant. It leaves you absolutely free to live every second just as it should be. No grasping or thinking that every bit has to be savoured; even that is gone.

Once you lose that aspect of time, of finiteness, you already are in contact with another world, with another sense of being. In the bed next to me was a very old lady, who had once been a school teacher. I'm sure she'd been a woman of great culture and education. She was upset often by the restrictions of hospital, of having to have the cot sides up on the bed, of not having control over her life at all, and especially of being strapped into the chair when she was allowed out of bed for a few hours in the morning. One morning, when she'd been crying over the captivity — it was actually the captivity of an old body, with the spirit really wishing to be free — I sat on the edge of the bed and I sang to her. She was fairly deaf and I knew she wouldn't hear the words, but I wanted her to hear the quality of what I was singing. And in a short time she was snoring her head off. I'm not sure whether that was an escape or whether in fact I had helped to salve her feelings. I longed to say to her "No one can take the freedom of your mind. Don't worry about the body, just live in your mind." But in fact it isn't your mind that lives on (that goes too) but the mind is the pathway to that other kind of being, that other kind of living that goes on.

By the time I was ready to come home I'd made some very strong contact with the nurses. And I'd been pleased to be able to use my homoeopathics there. I felt much easier about the prospect of my dying in that hospital. In fact once I'd loosed myself from the usual physical aspects of everyday life, death no longer seemed to have that explosive, terrible, final quality. I'd not been afraid of what happened after death, but of the actual dying: the slipping out of life had brought me disquiet. But now I can see that it's a quiet fading; dying in the way I am is a conscious sleep-taking journey, and each day a new place is achieved and each day I am closer.

Peter and I have worked a great deal on the pain aspect of my illness and last week I spoke to him of the pain in my shoulder blade which at times felt like a red hot knife. From that exploration I know that I have chosen to work through the pain, not to escape it, or deny it. When I do, nothing can ever touch me again. And it's only then that I'll really know what love is.

Easter is only a few days away and it now has a meaning that I never dreamed of. Last year I celebrated Easter as a time of sacred thought and Easter Sunday as a time of joy. But this time . . . for the first time I was achieving a small under-standing of the agony in the garden, and the meaning of Christ's death.

I am tentative, and feel great humility as I think of my entering the whole experience of Easter in a personal way.

It's interesting that I feel I know so much about the third-day experience, and from my regressive therapy I've known sudden and violent death. But now I was consciously entering into the pain of death and working through it, and with that I should understand that terrible agonizing death of Christ. When I was a child, and for almost all of my life I've tried to see the world as only a beautiful place, filled with love and constructive activity. During my therapy I've faced, worked through and discarded many destructive elements; and if I can penetrate the meaning of pain, if I can go through it and beyond it, some of the meaning of the world should come into focus. These thoughts are so elusive, and I'm still in the midst of working with them. I cannot write them for other people to know, for they are not things of the head, they are spheres for the whole being to enter into. My understanding is still slight and only beginning. As well as a sense of great contentment, overwhelming working, there's a feeling of joy, of looking forward to something beyond earthly conceiving.

I am comforted by the words of the Psalm beginning "I will lift up mine eyes unto the hills from whence does my help come." For in that Psalm it says that the Lord watches over our going out and our coming in. Interesting that it should be put in that order. I have a feeling often when I am deep in my meditation or prayer of a temple above me being prepared, like a great peak of wings, arcs of light, archways and pillars stretching up beyond my body endlessly. I feel safe and held by many things that I'm soon to know.

27. Easter

I still marvel at the pictures I have seen in my mind; pictures from past lives seemingly out of the ordinary sequence of time and yet there must have been some kind of pattern to them. It doesn't seem so important to me now to understand them exactly, especially since my experience this Easter. I can imagine someone reading my accounts and the conclusions I have come to, finding them very difficult to work with or to accept. It has not been easy for me; I must not shirk or deny what has come to me, for I did not seek it; I did not out of idle curiosity think it would be nice to try regressive therapy. It would also have been dishonest of me not to have included these experiences in my book, because they did happen to me, and whether or not others make the same sense of them as I have is their right. It has taken some courage to write about matters which many would consider to be delusions, silly ideas and in some cases, wicked ones. Whatever they have been, I have to be true to my own perception.

This week of Easter has been the culmination of a very long search, for no matter where I went in time or place, during these past three and a half years particularly, my search has been to understand the meaning of the shedding of the blood of Christ. I have sought to know and to see Christ at work, not in books or in the words of others, but in my own life. Christ didn't seem to me to be just a being to be apprehended when you walk through the door of death. He seemed to me to be a force which must light up everything that we do in our conscious life. That didn't just mean following the Ten Commandments or anything else that has been written or said by those who profess to know the truth. It meant going on a journey, similar to that of knights or of any others on their own personal search for the Holy Grail. At the beginning of Holy Week, I began reading the Gospel of St John and it seemed to me that if I were to understand the agony and pain of Christ's death, I would then fully understand two things. The most important is the great love that brought about the gift of his life for us — that is the gift of his shedding of blood on our behalf. The other, which is linked with it, is the taking on of responsibility for the darker side of life, for the cruelty, the pain and suffering which life has. If I could penetrate that agony in some way, to accept it and therefore go beyond it, then there would be nothing left but love. In a way, I would have overcome death as it appears to us at some stage in our lives. After that of course, nothing else could touch me.

Strange how so many people think of death as the end and yet for a very long time, if my experiences, my strange experiences, haven't done anything else, they have led me to a knowledge of life after death in a very tangible way. Death seems to me now a parting from the people I am presently with, and whom I am sure I will see again, but it is also a rebirth, a going into another state. I felt as if my death would be a quiet one, a kind of going into very deep prayer and not coming back.

As I read the Gospel of St John, I thought of that conscious wish of mine, to experience Christ's agony in a way to give me the understanding I was seeking. On Thursday, I woke with some pain and as the day progressed, it became worse and worse. The house was very busy with people coming and going, visitors and workmen, and Vivian read a Hermann Hesse book called *Wanderings* to me. I found it almost impossible to take my consciousness from my body and my pain, to the words of the book. I took analgesics, I had a hot bath, I tried hot water bottles and nothing I did touched the pain. It simply rose as if at will. At lunch time I took a stronger medicine and then I went into a kind of area of pain I'd never been in before. It was as though I were taken out of my body against my will. I clung on to my consciousness and tried to relax, but for an hour I felt as though I were truly drugged. To be drugged is to go to places outside your own travelling and your own will. Then the pain became a little fuzzier, but when Ben lifted me in and out of bed to use the pan, I felt as if all my bones were breaking. My friend Pat, who uses prayer a lot, happened to come into my room as Ben was laying me on the bed. I felt wretched and it seemed there was no place for me to go for peace or rest. The pain had undone me in a sense. I was crying as though my life was running out of me, as though my bones were breaking, as if my tongue were cloven to my mouth and as if death were close.

"Please go home," I asked Pat "and pray for me. I feel forsaken and I need strength," I did not have the strength to ask for it myself. During the afternoon, the crisis seemed to pass somewhat and the pain became a dull ache. I still felt very ill. That evening, Brian came and sat on the edge of my bed and in bold and confident tones, prayed with me that I might have relief from the pain and a good night's sleep. Thankfully, that's what I got.

Good Friday was a day of unreality but at least there was little pain. I had a kind of hangover from the previous day's events. I felt as though I'd been really wrung out. Early in the morning, because I could not read for myself, I turned on the radio to see if there was a Bible reading. A play, *The Eleventh of Twelve*, was in progress. I switched on to it just as they were portraying Christ on the cross, saying, "Father, why hast Thou forsaken me?" I was deeply shocked when the Roman soldier speared the side of Christ to see if he was still alive and my imagination did not need to work to understand the misery of the two, whose legs were broken to finish them off. As Christ's blood spilt to the earth, like the other bystanders in those ancient times, I almost felt it in my own heart. Up to that point, the experience of Christ's agony was one of the head, but with that shocking thrust and the spurting of water and blood, the experience moved right into the centre of my own heart, and so I understood that the pathway of blood from Christ to the earth is a pathway of tangible understanding for all of us. It is a reality that we can touch through the flowing of Christ's blood. I wonder if everyone at some time needs to penetrate that agony of dreadful physical death. As if in communion with the two who shared Christ's death on the cross, flanking him in his agony, I lost the use of my legs for about thirty-six hours. They felt shattered,quite frozen. I could not even lift my knees in the bed. Was the premonition I had voiced all those years ago, previous to my car accident, actually a voicing of the fear of my destiny — for now it is not my legs I am losing, but my life.

The following evening, I woke suddenly, not knowing why, ringing the bell and calling for Ben. It seemed that while I had been sleeping, I might have died. The possibility of sudden death came to my mind. It took me some time to think through that possibility, for I had come to expect with a deep certainty that my death would be a gentle flowing from one state of consciousness to another. I still have some things to do. I want to finish this book to the point where it can have a continuity even though it may still have blanks in the space of my life. I suppose it was during this time that I decided actually to ask for the strength and time to complete my book so that it may do its work.

The following day, Holy Saturday, was free from pain, a quiet day but very thoughtful, and then in the middle of the day I began to have an aching in my pelvis and my back, and quite unexpectedly, I began to menstruate. I had thought I would never menstruate again. I didn't know how long it was since the last time, for I seemed to have lost contact with that part of my existence. What did it mean? Again I was reminded of blood as the life-giving force, the carrier of regeneration, the support of new life — and so it seemed like the symbol of the river of life. My period only lasted for a little over 24 hours, as short by comparison as the remainder of my life perhaps. To end the Easter experience, Sunday was clear and still, a perfect day, full of peace and no hint of pain. There is no need for me to deny a word of my perception, or experience, for the meaning of my journey is that I have overcome, and am now prepared, for whatever pain I might have to endure. I will be prepared in the sense that I won't feel that I am forsaken, as I did last Thursday, ever again.

As I was going to sleep today, I asked for confirmation of my reality and for deep rest. I slept for three and a half hours in deep, untroubled sleep, the kind of rest I can look forward to when the battle finally finishes. I can see waiting for me all those wonderful women who have died in the past years from cancer. Women I have known for a short time and who have seemed to me to have been attending some purpose.

Now they seem to be soldiers for Christ in some way, not in the sense of aggressors, but soldiers in the sense of overcoming the power of death for us.

We must prepare ourselves for death. We cannot help but come to know Christ. I know that through this illness of mine and through my preparations, others have walked into the light as it were, and can see a positivity in what is happening. Their preparation through me is not by me, but from Christ. Every minute of this remaining life is Christ's and tonight as I listen to the rain after a long, dry summer and autumn, I feel the cleansing of the changing season and I look forward to the cleansing of the fire. I have been to Calvary in my own humble way. I have experienced in my own diluted way, as Brian pointed out, the words of Psalm 22:

> My God, my God, why has thou forsaken
>   me? . . .
> I am poured out like water,
>   and all my bones are out of joint;
> my heart is like wax,
>   it is melted within my breast;
> my strength is dried up like a potsherd,
>   and my tongue cleaves to my jaws;
>   thou dost lay me in the dust of death.

And now I will have some respite as I finish unfinished work. I realize that hospital was a very real preparation, for there I was separated from Ben and Kate and a step away from them. Hospital is an unreal sort of situation and so since I have come home, life has taken me up a little again. Once more, I feel the warmth of Ben's body next to me at night and I feel the strong threads of our ten years together and I listen with wonder at Kate's chatter and with joy to her singing. Inside me I have a feeling that seems akin to movements in deeper realms, of a majestically flowing river. Without summons, people I have known and shared my life with from years ago, are coming to say goodbye. The breath of eternal love moves to and from me. The reciprocal act of sharing with each other, is a breathing in and breathing out. The spirit is not some strange phenomenon which lives as a word in a book, or on the lips of someone behind a pulpit. I see it, I feel it, and I am a part of it and all the people who surround me with their warmth and care will feel it too. It is a living stream of creative energy, as ceaseless and as present as the wind, from which it draws its name. This world is a miraculous and beautiful creation, but what I have learnt and will soon experience, is regeneration, and that is the message of Easter. The ebb and flow of my life and my approaching death, is like a pendulum which moves in first one direction and then another, and finally, when the pendulum stops, all my focus will be together.

The world that I approach, I have seen recently in a meditation. I saw a most marvellous being with my mother in his arms. He moved gently through a perfect garden and then up towards an enormous range of hills. As he moved there, a great gust of breath took hold of us all, and swept us into the heights where we all reached a state of dreamless sleep. It was a state of timelessness and absolute harmony. As if the pendulum were still — not at rest, simply poised.

Now that I look back, many things have come into focus and much has been achieved. The lion of my dream has been slain and the giant whose footsteps echoed in my sleeping ears has been transformed into a being of great love and light. The two fears which stalked my unconscious mind, from the time I was a child; the two fears which I suppressed, but made manifest through physical illness and disquiet, have gone from me — the fear of calamitous event as symbolized by the lion and the actual fear of death as portrayed by the giant, have been vanquished.

A dream: my mother's voice

That sounds like my mother's voice. I was excited and pleased. She came into the room but did not greet me in the way a mother normally would. She stood there, young, beautiful and her essential self — vibrant with life, looking radiant.

"I've come," she said, "to make sure that you are absolutely certain that there is an after-life." My grandmother, a less distinct figure, sitting in profile to my left added, "Yes, and you will live again."

My Auntie Vera, completing the triangle, made a remark which indicated she believed all this to be true although she had not yet experienced it.

Poem

My feet move into the earth.
My toes move out like roots and tendrils,
seeking the nurture held in the earth.
My trunk is straight and tall.
My branches and all the growth of my life move
    towards heaven.
My tears blend with the rain,
my eyes are in the light,
and my breath flows with the wind.
My sap rises to expirate
and join with the stream of cosmic growth.
The seed of myself shapes and distils, poised —
ready to burst from its parent plant —
poised to journey forth into the air —
ready to find its place —
to sleep, to draw forth the riches of the soil
    of past life —
waiting to explode into new life when the time
    is ripe.
And where is my heart?
It lives in the warmth and the love
    of the eternal sun.

Postscript

Maxene had a clear vision of her book and the chapters were not written sequentially. Occasionally some of the names have been changed. Her methods of writing were various: she wrote in braille, she dictated on to casette tape, or directly to someone.

As the cancer overtook her, she became increasingly determined to complete the task. She finished it partially paralysed in bed at home, able to work on it for ten minutes at a time. Six weeks after the book was completed she died on September 8, 1982. She was forty-six.

Maxene saw clearly the need for a centre where different treatments and therapies were available, and so she became a founder of the Melbourne Therapy Centre for cancer and other patients.

Ben and Katie (now a teenager) still live in Melbourne. Ben is a teacher of Braille at the Royal Victoria Institute for the Blind. They enjoy each other's company, and have recently travelled overseas together, visiting some of the places Maxene mentions in her book.